P9-DFS-210

Fibromyalgia

and the
MindBodySpirit Connection

7 Steps for Living a Healthy Life
with Widespread Muscular Pain and Fatigue

William B. Salt II, M.D.
and
Edwin H. Season, M.D.

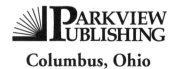

PARKVIEW PUBLISHING

Columbus, Ohio

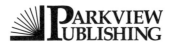

Parkview Publishing
P.O. Box 09784
Columbus, Ohio 43209-0784

Credits

Book interior design by Mary Ann Hopper
Cover design by Susan Sherron, Susan Edison, and Mary Ann Hopper
Photography by Susan Sherron, except Carol Gilbert: 141, 243
Illustrations by Shelley Salt, Kim Season, and Susan Sherron
Front and back cover photography © 1998 Susan Sherron

Copyright © 2000 William B. Salt II, M.D.
All rights reserved.
This book or any parts thereof may not be reproduced in any form or by any means, electronic or mechanical, including photocopying, recording, or by any information storage and retrieval system, without the written permission of the publisher.

ISBN 0-9657038-7-8
LC 99-66089

Warning

This book has been written and published in order to provide people with health information. It cannot serve as a substitute for consultation with a medical doctor. The information in this book is not the same as the practice of medicine and cannot replace or obviate consultation with a physician. The reader can choose, at his/her own risk, to act upon the knowledge and information presented herein. The authors and publisher recommend that the reader be aware of his/her health condition and status and consult a physician before beginning any health program, including changes in diet and undertaking an exercise plan.

Cataloging-in-Publication Data :

Salt, William Bradley, 1947-
    Fibromyalgia and the mindbodyspirit connection : 7 steps for living a healthy life with widespread muscular pain and fatigue / William B. Salt II and Edwin H. Season.
        p.   cm.
    Includes bibliographical references and index.
    ISBN 0-9657038-7-8
    1. Fibromyalgia--Popular works. I. Season, Edwin H. II. Title.
RC927.3.S35 1999   99-66089
616.7'4--DC 21   CIP

Printed by Malloy Lithographing, Inc.
Ann Arbor, Michigan, U.S.A.

Parkview Publishing Mission Statement

The mission of Parkview Publishing is to empower people who suffer from functional pain, symptoms, or syndromes (in which medical tests do not offer explanation) to heal and become healthier than ever before. This empowerment derives from knowledge, understanding, and acceptance of the following:

- State-of-the-art scientific medical diagnosis and treatment
- Interrelationships of *mind, body, spirit,* environment, and society

In order to achieve our mission, we at Parkview Publishing dedicate ourselves to the offering of empowering books, educational materials, resources, presentations, and a dynamic Web site, www.parkviewpub.com.

Background

There is an epidemic of unexplained symptoms, including widespread or localized bodily pain, fatigue, digestive complaints, headache, dizziness, chest pain, back pain, and gynecologic and urologic distress. Psychological symptoms, such as anxiety and depression, are often associated with them. All people suffer from some of these unexplained symptoms from time to time. When they become distressed with the symptoms, they consult with doctors who diagnose them as "functional" symptoms. The term "functional" means that even though the symptoms are very real, medical tests do not show an abnormality that accounts for them. Furthermore, collections of these symptoms are often diagnosed as functional syndromes, such as fibromyalgia and irritable bowel syndrome. These functional symptoms and syndromes can interfere greatly with one's quality of life and even the ability to carry out everyday activities and obligations, such as work.

Parkview Publishing offers a new language and way of understanding functional symptoms and syndromes. We consider functional symptoms to be *MindBodySpirit Symptoms* and functional syndromes to be *MindBodySpirit Syndromes*. The fact that various symptoms and syndromes occur together is evidence for a shared "cause" that can be understood through the interrelationships of *mind, body, spirit,* environment, and society.

MindBodySpirit Healing derives from understanding and appreciation of the *MindBodySpirit Connection,* the body's innate healing potential, the individual's responsibility for healing, distinctions between disease and illness and between treatment and healing, and the power of the patient-doctor/health professional relationship.

The MindBodySpirit Connection Series

Parkview Publishing is developing a series of books called the MindBodySpirit Connection Series. *Fibromyalgia and the MindBodySpirit Connection* is the second book, which follows *Irritable Bowel Syndrome & the Mind-Body/Brain-Gut Connection* (William B. Salt II, M.D., Columbus Ohio: Parkview Publishing, 1997). Currently in preparation are *Why Is My Stomach Hurting?* (a children's book) and a book addressing other functional *(MindBodySpirit)* symptoms and syndromes, including headache, fatigue, dizziness, back pain, chest pain, gynecologic/pelvic pain, and bladder and urinary symptoms.

Contents

INTRODUCTION

YOUR PRESCRIPTION FOR CHANGE!

We Have Your Prescription!

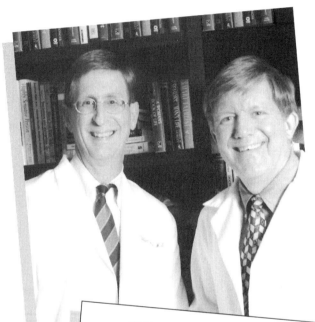

William B. Salt II, M.D. ◊ **Edwin H. Season, M.D.**

FOR   *YOU*

ADDRESS   *120 Elm Street, Anytown, USA*   DATE   *Today*

℞

LABEL WITH NAME OF MEDICATION

- Change your life forever.
- Don't allow fibromyalgia to control you.
- Discover the MindBodySpirit Connection.
- Understand the difference between disease and illness as well as the difference between treatment and healing.
- You have the power to heal and be well.
- Take the "medicine" from these pages and assume responsibility for your health.
- Use your fibromyalgia to turn the negative of illness into the positive of health!

William B. Salt II MD   *Edwin N Season MD*

REFILLS
0 • 1 • 2 • 3 • 4 • 5 • 1 YEAR

DEA No.   **1-888-599-6464**

Your Prescription for Change!

You always had it.
You always had the power.
– Glinda, the Good Witch in *The Wizard of Oz*

If you have unexplained *body* pain or have been diagnosed with fibromyalgia—or suspect that you might have fibromyalgia—then this book is for you. Furthermore, many people with certain types of arthritis, like osteoarthritis, and soft tissue rheumatic conditions also have fibromyalgia. If you have one or more of these conditions, then this book can help you too.

An Epidemic of Pain and Symptoms

There is an epidemic of musculoskeletal pain and discomfort in the Western countries, and the problem is getting worse. This pain involves the limbs of the body, the back, and the neck. Many patients with widespread *body* pain are diagnosed with what is called *fibromyalgia*. Disability from pain and fibromyalgia is increasing every year in American industry.

What Is Fibromyalgia?

Fibromyalgia is defined as widespread muscular aching, pain, and stiffness associated with tenderness on palpation (pressing the finger or thumb) on specified sites called trigger (tender) points located mainly in the neck, back, and extremities. These trigger or tender points are illustrated in Figure 1.

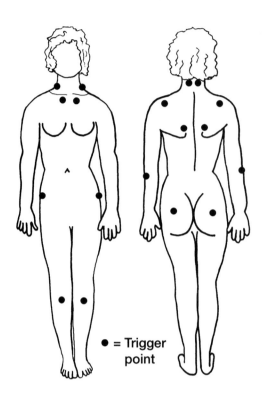

● = Trigger
       point

Figure 1

Other names for fibromyalgia include fibrositis, fibromyositis, and generalized myofascial pain. Table 1 shows that the pain of fibromyalgia is widespread.

Table 1		
Location of Pain in Fibromyalgia		
Base of skull	Chest	Legs
Neck	Back	Buttocks
Shoulders	Arms	Hips

What Is Myofascial Pain?

Myofascial pain syndrome is regional or localized fibromyalgia. Instead of being widespread, the pain and tenderness are found in a localized area of the body, the most common being the upper back, shoulders, and lower back. The muscles are very tender to any pressure, and nodules or lumps can often be felt within these muscles. The range of motion of nearby joints may also be limited.

Millions of People Are Affected

A study published recently in a medical journal indicates that fibromyalgia affects 2 percent of people in the United States. Fibromyalgia is ten times more common in women than in men. There is a progressive increase in the prevalence with age, such that about 7 percent of women 70 years of age are affected (*Arthritis and Rheumatism,* 1995).

Major Women's Health Problem

Most of the millions of Americans who suffer from fibromyalgia are women. Fibromyalgia is the most common cause of generalized musculo-skeletal pain in women between the ages of 20 and 55. Fibromyalgia is the second most common diagnosis made by rheumatologists. It is a major women's health issue and receives considerable media attention in newspapers, magazines, radio, and television.

Fibromyalgia: Worldwide Problem

Fibromyalgia has been described in most countries of the world. It does not appear to be related to ethnicity and is not a problem related to colder climates.

Fibromyalgia versus Arthritis

The muscles, tendons, ligaments, and joints are not inflamed in fibromyalgia as they can be in diseases like arthritis or myositis (inflamed muscles), so it is important to make the distinction with proper diagnosis. However, many people who do have these arthritic and inflammatory diseases also have fibromyalgia, so they too can benefit from the treatment advice offered in this book. Furthermore, it is a mistake to attribute the pain of fibromyalgia to coexisting arthritis or x-ray findings, and you will learn how this can interfere with healing.

Fibromyalgia: Consequences

Here are the consequences for many who suffer with fibromyalgia.

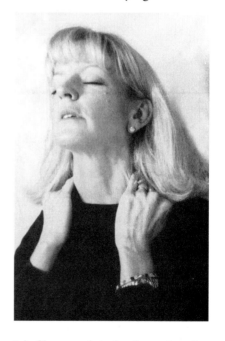

- Reduced sense of health and well-being
- Constant concerns related to the cause of the symptoms
- Sense of loss of control
- Reduced activity and exercise
- Difficulty with the activities of daily living
- Problems with interpersonal relationships with family, friends, and coworkers
- Disability with missed workdays

Fibromyalgia causes symptoms and discomfort ranging from mild and inconvenient to severe, resulting in incapacitation and disability. Current evidence shows that many patients with fibromyalgia lead restricted lives in multiple areas, including reduced physical activity, missed social opportunities, and lack of enjoyment of life. Many do not obtain much relief from current health care practices and medications.

So Many People with So Many Symptoms

Most people with fibromyalgia also have other unexplained symptoms, the most common of which are difficulty sleeping and fatigue. There is a virtual epidemic of *body* symptoms that have no apparent cause. In such cases, all of the tests—including physical examination, blood tests, x-rays, endoscopic examinations, and biopsy results—are normal. These symptoms that cause people to consult with doctors and that cannot be explained by tests are called "functional," "psychosomatic," or "somatization symptoms."

The symptoms listed in Table 2, including those of fibromyalgia, are the most common symptoms for which people consult with primary care doctors. Yet, a specific disease accounting for these symptoms can only be found in 10 percent to 20 percent of patients, or in one to two of every ten patients who consult with a doctor!

Table 2
Most Common *Body* Symptoms Are Functional (Tests Are Normal)

Fatigue and low energy *	Shortness of breath
Insomnia and difficulty sleeping *	Chest pain
Gastrointestinal (e.g., irritable bowel syndrome)	Abdominal pain and/or bowel problems
Headache	Back pain
TMJ pain (pain in the jaw)	Pelvic pain
Dizziness	Painful menstrual periods
Feeling faint	Decreased sex drive
Difficulty thinking and concentrating	Bladder problems

* The most common symptoms associated with fibromyalgia

People with Symptoms Become Patients with Functional Syndromes

Recognition of these "functional symptoms" leads to diagnosis with what doctors call "functional syndromes," or collections of symptoms that cannot be explained by medical science. People with functional symptoms who go to see a doctor become patients with functional syndromes. The main symptom and the type of doctor or specialist that a person sees usually determine the syndrome diagnosis that he or she first receives. As an

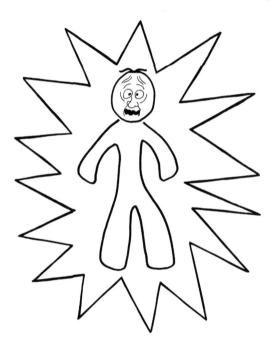

example, the rheumatologist diagnoses widespread musculoskeletal pain as **fibromyalgia;** the gastroenterologist diagnoses abdominal pain associated with bowel changes as **irritable bowel syndrome;** the dentist diagnoses jaw pain as **temporomandibular joint dysfunction;** the infectious disease expert may diagnose chronic fatigue and flu-like symptoms as **chronic fatigue syndrome (CFS);** the urologist diagnoses difficulties with urination as **irritable bladder syndrome** or **interstitial cystitis;** and the gynecologist diagnoses pelvic discomfort and pain as **chronic pelvic pain syndrome.**

Are These Symptoms and Syndromes "All in the Head"?

Unfortunately, terms like "functional," "psychosomatic," and "somatization" are often interpreted to suggest that the symptoms are "all in the head," phoney, or imagined. The truth is that the symptoms are very real. In fact, virtually everyone experiences one or more functional symptoms (or syndromes if diagnosed by a doctor) from time to time. However, some people have symptoms that are frequent, constant, and severe, which causes them to consult with doctors. The suffering is enormous; it is personal, social, and economic.

What is going on here? What is the common denominator? The answer is that the problem is not "all in the head" but is related to the connection between the brain *(mind)* and *body.*

The MindBodySpirit Connection

You will learn that *mind* and *body* are one. It no longer makes sense to classify problems as either stress/emotional related *(mind)* or physical *(body).* Furthermore, you will discover why it is essential that the *mind-body* connection include *spirit;* scientific evidence continues to confirm the mysterious power of *spirit* and how affirming beliefs—particularly belief in a higher power—can contribute signifi-cantly to health.

You will study the neurochemical basis of the *mind-body-spirit* connec-tion. You will learn that there are three systems of communication.

We will propose a new lan-guage in this book for people with functional symptoms, patients with functional syn-dromes, and the doctors who diagnose them. The four new terms that we will introduce are the following:

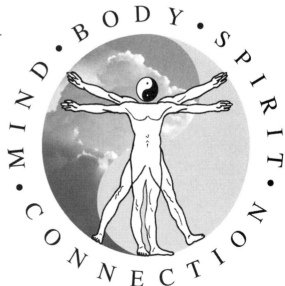

- *MindBodySpirit Connection*
- *MindBodySpirit Symptoms*
- *MindBodySpirit Syndromes*
- *MindBodySpirit Healing*

You will appreciate that *MindBodySpirit Healing* is based upon the recognition and acceptance of the connection between *mind, body,* and *spirit,* the distinction between treatment and healing, the innate healing potential of the *body,* and the power of the partnership between the patient and doctor/health professional in restoring health.

You will understand fibromyalgia as a *MindBodySpirit Syndrome,* which is a collection of *MindBodySpirit Symptoms.* You will better appreciate the "cause" of fibromyalgia by understanding the biopsychosocial-spiritual model, the *MindBodySpirit Connection,* and systems thinking.

Why a Book about Fibromyalgia?

There have been new developments in the diagnosis and treatment of fibromyalgia and other soft tissue rheumatic disorders. Furthermore, everyone (people with symptoms, patients with syndromes, and doctors who diagnose them) can become more aware of a person's ability to heal from *MindBodySpirit Symptoms* and *MindBodySpirit Syndromes* by understanding the *MindBody-Spirit Connection* and leading a healthy lifestyle.

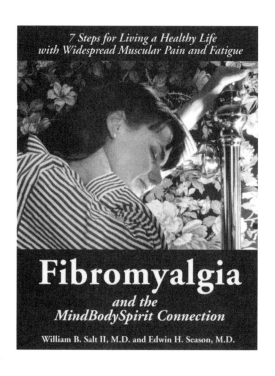

The impact of "managed care" means that your doctor will have less time to spend with you. In fact, most doctor visits are now limited to 12 minutes or less! This does not leave much time for diagnosis, education, and treatment. It may also be difficult and expensive for you to see a specialist because the managed care system expects that your primary care physician should be able to handle most problems.

The model of interaction between patient and physician is changing. YOU are given more responsibility in the management of your own care. You will need and must have accurate and reliable information in order to fulfill this personal responsibility and opportunity.

The Power of Knowledge

You gain the upper hand by understanding the *MindBodySpirit Connection* and by an appreciation of the impact of perceived stress, emotional distress, thought, and memory on the conscious and unconscious *mind, body,* and *spirit.* Just knowing the "cause" of fibromyalgia is beneficial. Focusing on the power of your *mind* rather than on the pain and diagnosis of your *body* can bring lifelong relief.

With this book, you can explore your diagnostic and treatment options in the privacy of your home and on your own time. Then, armed with information and knowledge about your problem, you will be better able to partner with your doctor in order to heal.

You Can Heal!

Your *mind, body,* and *spirit* are connected and inseparable. You will learn that you are stronger than you ever thought and that you have more control over your *body* than you realized. The goal of this book is to show you that the illness of fibromyalgia is a *MindBodySpirit Syndrome* and to provide the tools for you to access the miraculous ability of your *body* to heal through the *MindBodySpirit Connection.* Furthermore, your problem can be the stimulus for a life change that will bring you better health and wellness than you have had before.

Learn to Be Healthy

You can learn to be healthy. Accurate information leads to healing and is often much more important than medication. Achieving health and wellness is an active, rather than passive, process. The focused information on fibromyalgia in this book is integrated with holistic *MindBodySpirit Connection* concepts and the latest information on living a healthy lifestyle.

It may take you up to twelve weeks to read this book and walk through the seven steps listed in Table 3. Change is never easy, but then neither is it easy to live with fibromyalgia. Behavioral psychologists have studied people who have succeeded in changing their lives. Research shows that it takes about 12 weeks to make the commitment, begin to change behavior, and to establish an enduring life change.

Table 3

7 Steps for Living a Healthy Life with Fibromyalgia

Step 1: Connecting Mind, Body, and Spirit
Step 2: Learning about Fibromyalgia and Myofascial Pain
Step 3: Healing with Diagnosis and Education
Step 4: Making "The Connection"
Step 5: Emphasizing Self-Care and Wellness
Step 6: Managing Your Fibromyalgia
Step 7: Taking Action If Symptoms Persist

"Use" Fibromyalgia

Not only can you heal from fibromyalgia, but also you can be healthier than you have ever been. Turn the negative of your illness into the positive of health and wellness. You can "use" fibromyalgia to change your life and health.

Focus on the power of your mind rather than on the pain of your body. Use the diagnosis of fibromyalgia to realize your ability to heal through the MindBodySpirit Connection and become healthier than ever before.

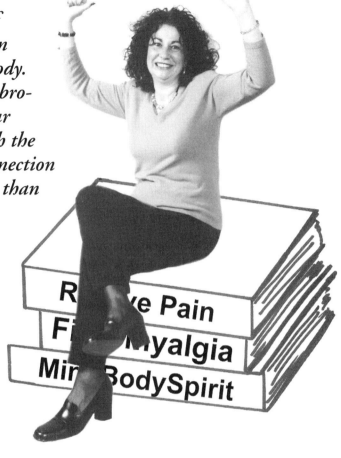

R...ve Pain
Fi...Myalgia
Min...BodySpirit

Welcome to wellness!

William B. Salt II MD

William B. Salt II, M.D.
Gastroenterologist
Author of *Irritable Bowel Syndrome & The Mind-Body/Brain-Gut Connection*
Columbus, Ohio

Edwin H. Season MD

Edwin H. Season, M.D.
Orthopedic Surgeon
Columbus, Ohio

STEP 1

CONNECTING MIND, BODY, AND SPIRIT

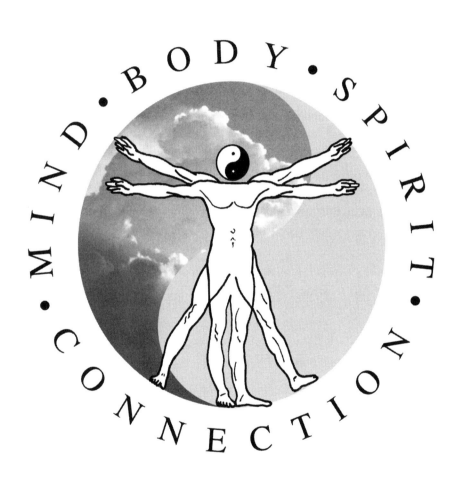

MIND · BODY · SPIRIT · CONNECTION

Chapter 1
Body

. . . the first stage of healing always begins with breakdown. The first stage of healing is characterized by a focus on, and attention to, the external manifestations of distress (symptoms).

– Intentional Healing
Elliott Dacher, M.D.

When my brother died in 1966, my father began a grieving process that lasted almost twenty-five years. For all that time he suffered from chronic, debilitating headaches. I took him to some of the country's major medical facilities, but no one could cure him of his pain. At one point, during that ongoing search for help, a doctor tried to teach him that his headaches were somehow related to his grief. But my father persisted in treating his pain exclusively as a medical problem, and the headaches continued to torment him.

– Healing and the Mind
Bill Moyers

There is an epidemic of unexplained *body* pain and symptoms, and everyone experiences them—including the authors of this book!

Normal Body Feelings: Here Today, Gone Tomorrow

Pain can be anywhere and can last for moments to days, but it eventually goes away. Sometimes excess physical work or unaccustomed exercise accounts for it. Other times the pain seems to be associated with a stress in life. Mostly though, the pain seems to have a *mind* of its own. It is a mystery as to how it starts and how it stops.

Dr. Lewis Thomas described this reality in his book, *Lives of a Cell* (New York: Penguin, 1995), when he said, "The great secret, known to internists and learned early in the marriage by internists' wives, but still hidden from the general public, is the fact that most things get better by themselves. Most things, in fact, are better by morning."

Not Gone Tomorrow

Most people also experience symptoms that are more troublesome because they are more intense and/or last longer. The pain may be in the neck and shoulder or upper or middle back. Pain can involve the joints: shoulders, elbows, wrists, fingers, hips, knees, ankles, and/or feet.

Let's talk about you. The pain may be worse during either the day or the night. It may be more severe when you first get out of bed and may improve as the day goes on. By contrast, the pain may become progressively severe as the day wears on. Pain may be either improved or aggravated by standing, walking, or sitting. Or the pain may occur at totally unpredictable times and not occur when you expect it to.

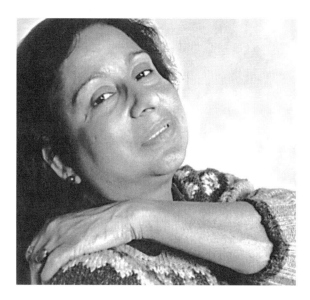

You may fear certain activities and positions and be afraid to lift anything or bend over. The pain, avoidance of activities, and fear can interfere with your ability to do your job or work at home. You may no longer exercise or participate in sports because of the pain and fear. Or if you still play, you do so in spite of the pain.

Pain can last for days, weeks, months, or years. It may be recurrent, and it may have started with an accident or injury. Sometimes you are aware that you are under stress, anxious, or depressed; sometimes you are not able to pinpoint any correlation or reason.

The Doctor, the Tests

If you go to the doctor with the concern that something is wrong, one of two things happens: either the tests are completely normal, or something shows up on the evaluation. The physical examination may show that it hurts when the doctor presses on certain parts of your body: the top of the shoulders, the small of the back, the outer part of the buttock, or the outside of the thighs. If the pain is localized, then a diagnosis of tendonitis, a muscle strain, tear, "pull," or **myofascial pain** may be made. If it is generalized, you have probably been told that you have **fibromyalgia.**

If x-rays, CT scan, or MRI are ordered, they are most likely normal. However, they might show a bone spur, torn cartilage, a deteriorating or degenerating spine, a bulging disk, or "arthritis." The pain gets worse if you learn or believe that it could be related to the diagnosis or the finding on the tests, even though the reality is that the findings are not the cause of the pain. When the pain continues, you consult with other doctors and specialists. Even if it gets better for a while, the pain always comes back.

Pain and Symptoms Domination

The pain may dominate your life, remaining constantly with you and in your thoughts. It can sap your energy, interfere with sleep, and become associated with anxiety, depression, or both. You may live your life around the symptoms and illness.

Body Pain and Symptoms

These very real physical symptoms and pain that cannot be explained by tests occur in everyone from time to time. Many people consult doctors when the symptoms are considered bothersome, raise concerns about a serious disease, and/or interfere with life's activities, including work. Doctors refer to these symptoms as "functional," "psychosomatic," or "somatization" symptoms. We don't like the terms. They carry a negative connotation and seem to most people to mean that the pain is phoney or imagined. This is one reason why we will propose a new terminology in Chapter 8. These *body* symptoms which cannot be explained by tests are part of the evidence that the *body* and *mind* are connected.

In the next chapter, you will learn about this amazing *mind-body* connection.

Chapter 2
Mind-Body

This is Descartes' error: the abysmal separation between body and mind . . . the suggestion that reasoning, and moral judgment, and the suffering that comes from physical pain or emotional upheaval might exist separately from the body. Specifically: the separation of the most refined operations of the mind from the structure and operation of a biological organism.

– *Descartes' Error*
Dr. Antonio R. Damasio

The *mind* (brain) is connected to the *body.* This is easy to demonstrate by the muscle tension, sweating, rapid heartbeat, and shortness of breath that can occur with any anxiety-provoking situation.

Mind and Body Are Connected

People differ in what emotions or body sensations they feel and whether they are more or less aware of what is occurring in the *mind* and *body.* Some are more sensitive to signals that the *body* sends to the brain. It is normal to have *mind-body* symptoms; everyone has them. Many of us can associate these symptoms with stress and emotion.

Do you remember . . .
- That stiff neck or back in the morning when you were overwhelmed with work?
- That funny feeling in your stomach when you first fell in love?
- The "butterflies" before the big games?
- The nausea and upset stomach before giving a speech?
- The cramps and diarrhea before your big job interview?

Memory is important. Perhaps you can experience *body* symptoms now when you recall something that was associated with stress and/or emotion. Think back to something either extremely exciting or embarrassing. You may actually be able to feel those same symptoms just by the memory of the experience. The relationship of *body* symptoms and *mind* relative to conscious and unconscious stress, emotional distress, thought, and memory is further evidence of the power of the *mind-body* connection.

Understanding the *mind-body* connection is the key to healing with fibromyalgia. To begin your journey, first look at the difference between disease and illness.

The Difference between Disease and Illness: Sam, Sharon, and Shelley

A **disease** is an identifiable abnormality of the body that can be verified by testing. An **illness** is a person's perception of ill health. There can be a remarkable discordance between **disease** and **illness** because they are not the same. Look at Figure 2.1 where you will meet Sam, Sharon, and Shelley.

Disease, Illness, or Both?

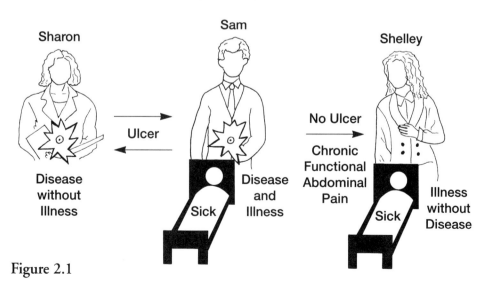

Sharon

Sam

Shelley

Ulcer

No Ulcer

Chronic Functional Abdominal Pain

Disease without Illness

Disease and Illness

Illness without Disease

Sick

Sick

Figure 2.1

You see that both Sam and Sharon have identical stomach ulcers that were discovered when they underwent stomach testing during a research project. The ulcer is a **disease.** It is a definable abnormality that doctors can detect and identify.

Sam has so much abdominal pain associated with his ulcer that he is sick and missing work. Sam has a **disease and illness.**

By contrast, Sharon has no symptoms whatsoever even though she has an ulcer in her stomach (it is quite common for people to have ulcers without having symptoms). Sharon has a **disease without illness.**

Now look at Shelley. She has abdominal pain, but there is no ulcer in her stomach. Tests do not show a scientific and medical cause for her abdominal pain even though it is real and not imagined. Shelley has an **illness without disease.** She has what doctors call "chronic functional abdominal pain."

Fibromyalgia: An Illness without Disease

Fibromyalgia is associated with pain and fatigue even though tests show no identifiable abnormalities. Fibromyalgia is another example of illness without disease. There is nothing phoney or imaginary about the symptoms of an illness without disease like chronic functional abdominal pain and fibromyalgia. The pain and fatigue are very real indeed.

Illness without Disease: Functional Body Symptoms

Many who have fibromyalgia also have other unexplained symptoms, the most common of which are difficulty sleeping and fatigue. The symptoms listed in Table 2 of the introductory chapter, *Your Prescription for Change!,* along with the pain and fatigue of fibromyalgia, are the most common symptoms that cause people to see primary care doctors. Yet, a specific disease accounting for these symptoms can only be found in 10 percent to 20 percent of patients, or one to two of every ten patients who consult with a doctor! Here again is **illness without disease.**

Doctors call these symptoms "functional," "psychosomatic," or "somatization" symptoms because they are not explained by medical tests. These terms have assumed a somewhat negative connotation; they suggest that the symptoms are phoney or imagined. In Chapter 17, you will discover how functional symptoms that cause people to see doctors are diagnosed as functional syndromes (like fibromyalgia), which are collections of functional symptoms. People with symptoms become patients with syndromes. In Chapter 8, we will introduce a new terminology that will help people with symptoms, patients with syndromes, and doctors who diagnose them to communicate with a shared and positive language.

The Mind-Body Connection: The First Step to Healing

The phenomenon of **illness without disease,** or symptoms without medical basis, cannot be understood without understanding the *mind-body* connection and what doctors call the biopsychosocial model of disease and illness.

Functional body pain and symptoms affect so many different body systems and parts because there is an alteration or abnormality in the way that the *mind* (brain) processes pain and sensation, which results in increased *mind* sensitivity to *body* signals. This will be discussed in Chapters 4 and 5.

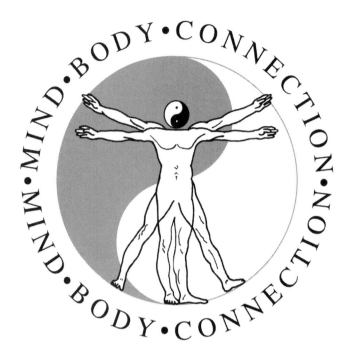

Perceived stress, emotional distress, thought, and memory are very important. They affect and influence whether and to what extent and degree people experience symptoms, whether they feel ill with them, whether they will miss work or social opportunities, and whether they will report them to doctors.

The *mind-body* connection is critical to understanding not only fibromyalgia, but also all human disease and illness. Understanding this connection is central to self-care, the achievement of health and wellness, and healing.

The Mind-Body Relationship: A Brief History

Throughout history, philosophers have considered two different views: first, that the *mind* and *body* are part of the same system; second, that they are entirely separate. As Harvard's Herbert Benson, M.D., has said,

"A review of ancient history shows that we are returning to original beliefs that the mind and body cannot be separated" (*Timeless Healing: The Power and Biology of Belief*, New York: Scribner, 1996).

Most evidence suggests that the *mind* and *body* were considered as a unit by the ancient cultures (Taylor, Shelley, *Health Psychology*, New York: McGraw-Hill, Inc., 1995). People believed that evil spirits entered the body and caused disease and that health could be restored by exorcising and removing these spirits from the *body*. Later, the Greeks attributed disease to *body* factors (the humoral theory of illness) but believed that these factors could also affect the *mind*. They proposed the concept of "Holos," that medical disease involved the whole person instead of only the diseased *body* part. This is the view that is held by many non-Western societies.

The pendulum swung back toward mental explanations for illness during the Middle Ages. Disease and illness were felt to be God's punishment for evil doing. Cure was often sought by torturing the body to drive out evil. Later, this "treatment" was replaced by penance achieved through prayer and good works.

The Renaissance brought progressive understanding of the human *body* and disease based upon scientific discovery and technology, such as the microscope. As a result of these advances, medicine turned more and more to scientific investigation of the *body* rather than the *mind* as the basis for medical progress. Great emphasis was placed upon the dualistic concept of *mind* and *body* in order to break with superstition of the past.

In 1637, the French philosopher and mathematician, René Descartes, was the first to suggest that the body did not require the mind to operate. For the next 300 years, physicians emphasized that abnormalities at the cellular level and organic disorders were the sole cause of illness and disease. Physical evidence became the only basis for diagnosis and treatment of illness. This is known as the **biomedical model** of health, disease, and illness.

The concept that physical health is integrated with the psychological and social environment evolved from the work of Sigmund Freud and the rise of modern psychiatry. In the late 1970s, George Engel proposed the **biopsychosocial model** of health, disease, and illness.

The Biomedical Model versus the Biopsychosocial Model

The **biomedical model** has governed the thinking of most health practitioners for the past 300 years. It holds that all illness can be explained based upon disorder and disease of body anatomy and processes—that is, biologically. It assumes that psychological and social processes are mainly independent of the disease process. The **biomedical model** reflects *mind-body* dualism with the *mind* and the *body* as separate entities. It emphasizes illness over health rather than health over illness.

By contrast, the **biopsychosocial model** of health, disease, and illness holds that the biological, psychological, and social factors are all interrelated elements of health and illness. For example, the presence or absence of social support, high levels of stress, depression, and disorders or chemical imbalances at a cellular level all interact to produce a state of health or illness. Health and illness are caused by multiple factors and produce multiple effects. The *mind* and *body* cannot be separated in relation to issues of health and illness because they both influence the state of health. The **biopsychosocial model** emphasizes both health and illness, rather than considering illness to be a deviation from some healthy state.

The implication of this for you is that achieving health is an active process rather than a passive one. Understanding the *mind-body* connection is essential. You must attend to your biological, psychological, and social needs.

Through the "Lens" of the Biopsychosocial "Camera"

Fibromyalgia and other unexplained bodily symptoms cannot be understood without looking through the "lens" of the **biopsychosocial** "camera." You have a responsibility to focus upon your own health. "Picture" yourself healthy!

Back to Sam, Sharon, and Shelley

Although Sam and Sharon have the same disease, only Sam is ill. Sharon has good health habits, manages stress, and feels good about herself. She does not feel her ulcer. It may also be that her *body* (stomach) is not as sensitive as Sam's is. Differences in *body* sensitivity may be both biological (genetic or inherited) and psychosocial (learned).

Suppose Sam has always had a low pain threshold and frequent stomachaches. As a child, his mother allowed him to miss school frequently for abdominal pain and illness. He saw a doctor frequently because both he and his mother tended to think the worst about the possible explanations for his symptoms. Neither one appreciated any relationship between stress and symptoms. He is under great stress and does not take good care of himself. In fact, he is depressed. He is ill with the pain of the ulcer.

It should be easier to see how real pain and symptoms can occur in an individual who has an illness without disease like Shelley with chronic functional abdominal pain. Fibromyalgia is very much like chronic functional abdominal pain. It is an illness without disease.

Once you understand the *mind-body* connection, you can learn how to relieve your symptoms and heal. You have more control over your *body* with your *mind* than you may realize.

The next chapter addresses the remarkable and accumulating evidence of the importance of spirituality relative to health and wellness.

Chapter 3
Mind-Body-Spirit

Rest, rest perturbed spirit.
– Hamlet (1601)
William Shakespeare

Religion confronts the individual with the most momentous option life can present. It calls the soul to the highest adventure it can undertake: the call to confront reality and master the self. The enduring religions at their best contain the distilled wisdom of the human race.
– Huston Smith
(author of *The World's Religions*)
from *The Wisdom of Faith with Huston Smith: A Bill Moyers Special*

The healing power of faith is not a new idea, but scientific studies are increasingly documenting the health benefits of spirituality and religion. As an example, persons who attended religious services had significantly lower mortality than those who did not attend (*American Journal of Public Health* 88:1469, 1998).

Mind-Body

Mind-body medicine refers to the concept that thoughts and emotions have a significant impact on the health of the *body* as well as the prevention and treatment of disease and illness. There is a renewed interest in this ancient model because of increasing emphasis by the public, new scientific understanding of the chemistry of *mind-body* communication, and demonstration of medical value of several *mind-body* approaches.

Researchers at Harvard Medical School have been studying the benefits of *mind-body* interactions for more than 25 years. They have shown that when a person engages in a repetitive prayer, word, sound, or phrase and when intrusive thoughts are passively disregarded, a specific set of physiologic changes ensues. In what Harvard's Dr. Herbert Benson calls the "relaxation response" (Chapter 21), there is slowing of metabolism, heart rate, rate of breathing, and brain waves. These changes are opposite of those brought about by stress and are an effective treatment for numerous diseases and illnesses, including hypertension, irregularities of heart rhythm, many forms of chronic pain, insomnia, infertility, symptoms of cancer and AIDS, premenstrual syndrome, anxiety, and mild to moderate depression. Any illness or disease that is either caused or made worse by stress may benefit by these physiologic changes.

Mind-Body-Spirit

Harvard research has also established that people who elicited the "relaxation response" experienced a sense of increased spirituality regardless of whether or not they utilized a repetitive focus. Spirituality is the experience of the presence of a power, force, energy, or perception of God. This presence was perceived as close to the person. Importantly, spirituality was associated with fewer medical symptoms.

In 1910, Sir William Osler, perhaps the most well-known physician and proponent of modern scientific medicine of his time, wrote of "the faith that heals." Dr. Benson believes that we are all "wired for God" and that spirituality and religious faith enhance healing through the placebo effect, or what he calls, "remembered wellness." This will be further explored in Chapters 12–14.

The intuition, experience, and scientific research attesting to the healing power of spirituality, faith, and prayer are the reasons that the concept of the *mind-body* connection should be expanded to include *spirit*. Thus, the more appropriate term is the *mind-body-spirit* connection.

The Biopsychosocialspiritual Model

You learned about the biopsychosocial model of health, illness, and disease in the last chapter. We propose that this is medical professional language for the *mind-body* connection.

The spirituality of patients is being brought to the mainstream of medical education, research, and care. Three years ago, only three medical schools offered courses on religion and spiritual issues. Today, more than 30 medical schools offer such courses. The National Institutes of Health (NIH) has funded research to investigate religion as a determinant of physical and mental health and has sponsored recent conferences called Methodological Approaches to the Study of Religion, Health, and Aging and Spiritual Assessment in Health Care Settings. It seems appropriate then, that a more inclusive term to describe the relationship of *mind, body,* and *spirit* is the biopsychosocialspiritual model. Furthermore, we propose that this is medical professional language for the *mind-body-spirit* connection.

Healing and Spirit

Recent researchers and authors have been emphasizing the healing power and potential of faith, spirituality, belief in a higher power, and prayer. Evidence is accumulating that the value of spirituality in healing and maintaining health has been greatly underestimated.

The following are several outstanding resources relative to the significance of spirituality and religion in healing.

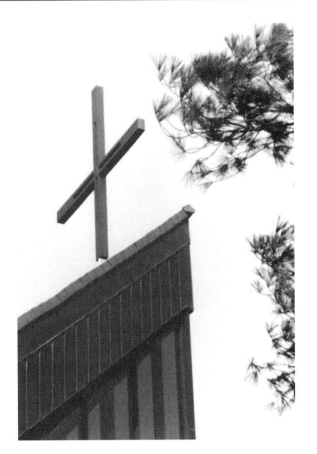

- "Emperor of the Soul," *Time* magazine, by David Van Biema, June 24, 1996, pp. 65–68.

- "Faith & Healing," *Time* magazine, by Claudia Wallis, June 24, 1996, pp. 58–64.

- *Healing Words: The Power of Prayer and the Practice of Medicine,* (New York: Harper Collins, 1993) by Larry Dossey, M.D., an internal medicine specialist who now writes on a full-time basis about spirituality and healing.

- *It's Better to Believe: The New Medical Program That Uses Spiritual Motivation to Achieve Maximum Health and Add Years to Your Life,* (Nashville: Thomas Nelson, Inc. 1995), by Kenneth H. Cooper, M.D., the doctor who made "aerobics" a household word.

- "Religion and Spirituality in Medicine: Research and Education," *Journal of the American Medical Association* by Levin, Larson, and Puchalski, September 3, 1997, pp. 792–793.

- *The Road Less Traveled: A New Psychology of Love, Traditional Values, and Spiritual Growth,* (New York: Touchstone, 1978), by M. Scott Peck, M.D., who has been integrating psychology, spirituality, science, and health for many years.

- *Science and Health with Key to the Scriptures,* (Boston: The First Church of Christ, Scientist, 1994), by Mary Baker Eddy, founder of Christian Science and first published in 1875.

- *Timeless Healing: The Power and Biology of Belief,* (New York: Scribner, 1996) by Herbert Benson, M.D., (with Marg Stark) of Harvard's Mind/Body Medical Institute who described the Relaxation Response.

You are now prepared to explore the connection of *mind, body,* and *spirit* in the next chapter.

Chapter 4

The Mind-Body-Spirit Connection

If we're to understand what role our emotions may play
in our health, then understanding the molecular-cellular
domain is the crucial first step.
– Molecules of Emotion
Dr. Candace Pert (Neuroscientist)

Buddhists have a wonderful term for our churning mental chaos:
"monkey mind." Like monkeys jumping from tree limb to tree limb,
our minds often leap from thought to thought with little reprieve.
When one has a monkey mind, excessive brain activity can overload
the system, making it difficult to concentrate, to learn new things,
and to fall asleep. Because they are repeatedly instructed to do so,
your muscles will also eventually clench out of habit, not just in
stressful situations. This muscle tension sends a distress signal to
the brain, perpetuating a vicious cycle of physical mobilization for
the sake of physical mobilization without relief in sight.
– Timeless Healing
Herbert Benson, M.D.

There is a connection of *mind* and *body* through three systems of
communication (and possibly a fourth). By understanding the science of this connection, you have more power over your *body* and
fibromyalgia symptoms than you may think.

Science and the Mystery of Spirit

In this chapter, you will come to understand the scientific basis for how
the *mind* and *body* communicate with one another through the *mind-body*
connection. Healing comes through understanding. However, Chapter 3

introduced some of the evidence for the mystifying healing power of belief, faith, and *spirit*. We have included *spirit* in the title of this chapter in order to emphasize that the scientific connection of *mind-body* is also embedded within, and connected to, the mystery of the *spirit*. Hereafter in this book, we will refer to the *mind-body* connection as the *mind-body-spirit* connection.

Psychoneuroimmunology: Beliefs to Reality

There is a new field of medical investigation called psychoneuroimmunology (PNI), which integrates the studies of the *mind* (psychology), the brain (neurology), and the immune system, or the natural healing system of the *body* (immunology). In Chapter 2, you learned that beliefs about the *mind-body* relationship have varied throughout recorded history. Psychiatric medicine emerged in the early 1900s and proposed that mental disorders could give rise to physical disorders. Later, psychosocial research into the relationship of emotional distress to illness and disease advanced the concept of a *mind-body* relationship. Finally, PNI has emerged as a highly disciplined field of scientific inquiry that is confirming the nature of the *mind-body-spirit* connection. Beliefs have become reality.

The Role of the Brain

The brain plays a central role in translating the content of the *mind*—perceptions, thoughts, attitude, emotion, and memory—into nerve impulses and biochemistry. For simplicity, we will use the terms "brain" and *"mind"* interchangeably. The *mind* communicates with the *body* via a connection through the central nervous system, the autonomic nervous system, and the neuropeptide chemical messenger system. Information travels in both directions: *mind* to *body, body* to *mind.*

Let's take a closer look at the three communication systems of the *mind-body-spirit* connection (Figure 4.1).

Three Communication Systems

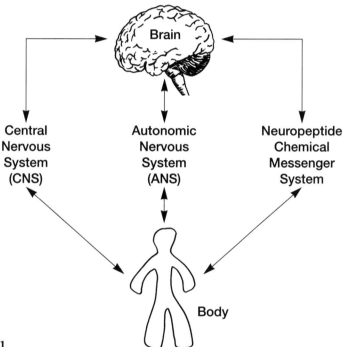

Figure 4.1

The Central Nervous System (CNS)

The central nervous system, called the CNS, is composed of the brain and the spinal cord. The nerves to the skeletal muscles run directly from the CNS. This nervous system translates the intention to move a muscle into electrical nerve impulses that result in movement of the *body.*

The Autonomic Nervous System (ANS)

The autonomic nervous system, or ANS, includes two main branches that emanate from the spinal cord. They control the involuntary or unconscious action of the glands and the smooth muscle of the heart, blood vessels, and intestinal tract (Figure 4.2). These two branches of the autonomic nervous system act in opposition to each other. You will learn that these involuntary or unconscious systems can be consciously controlled.

Autonomic Nervous System (ANS)

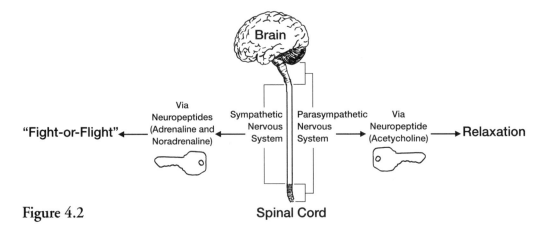

Figure 4.2

The sympathetic branch

One branch of the autonomic nervous system is called the sympathetic branch, and the nerves that control it are located in the thoracic (chest) and lumbar (lower back) segments of the spinal cord. The sympathetic branch uses the neuropeptides adrenaline and noradrenaline to activate the "fight-or-flight" stress reaction in emergencies. Neuropeptides are discussed later in this chapter, and the "fight-or-flight" stress response is explored in Chapter 5.

The parasympathetic branch

The other branch of the autonomic nervous system is called the parasympathetic branch, which is located in the cranial (top) and sacral (bottom) segments of the spinal cord and uses the neuropeptide acetylcholine to relax the body. In general, the parasympathetic branch induces relaxation, which is the opposite reaction of the "fight-or-flight" response. For example, the lowering of the heart rate and blood pressure and the reduction of muscle tension are produced by the parasympathetic branch. As you will learn, all stress management techniques aim to induce a positive parasympathetic state (Chapters 5 and 21).

The Neuropeptide Chemical Messenger System

The most recently discovered system that connects *mind* and *body* is the neuropeptide chemical messenger system. In order to appreciate this amazing system, you need to understand some basic biologic concepts.

Basic science

You have sensory organs with which you scan your world: your eyes, ears, nose, tongue, and skin. All cells of your *mind* and *body* have thousands of locations on their surface that serve as sensors on a cellular level. These are called **receptors.** See Figure 4.3(a). Think of each receptor as a **lock.** It is waiting to receive a chemical messenger called a **neuropeptide.** See Figure 4.3(b). Think of a neuropeptide as a **key** that can enter the keyhole of the receptor lock. The message of the neuropeptide is transmitted to the receptor, which then transmits it from the surface of the cell into the interior of the cell.

Neuropeptide Chemical Messenger System

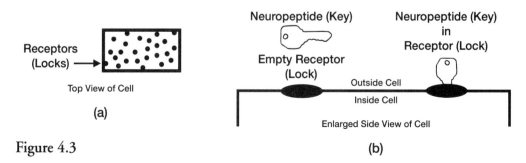

Figure 4.3

23

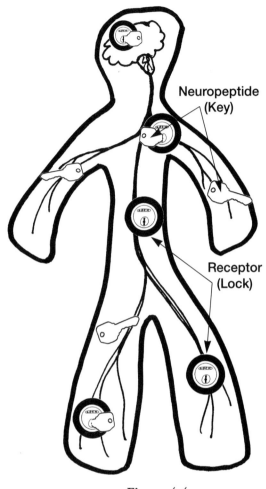

Neuropeptide
(Key)

Receptor
(Lock)

Figure 4.4

Figure 4.4 illustrates this neuropeptide communication system, which is found throughout your *mind* and *body*. The neuropeptides (keys) float in the fluid that surrounds the cells containing the receptors (locks). Note that not all receptors are occupied by neuropeptides because receptors ignore all but the particular type of neuropeptide made to fit it.

Molecules of emotion

Dr. Candace Pert, a neuroscientist and researcher, has done extensive work in the biochemistry of emotions and in the field of psychoneuroimmunology, which is the study of the relationship between psychological factors and the nervous and immune systems. Her studies of these neuropeptides and their receptors show that there is a network in which all types of information, including emotional information, is circulated throughout the mind and *body*. This network allows organs and systems to influence and affect one another (*Molecules of Emotion*. New York: Scribner, 1997).

Messages and symptoms coming from one location in your body can affect many other locations. The *mind* can upset the *body*. This is how stress, thought, emotion, and psychological problems can affect bodily sensation and function. You can see how a fight with your spouse can cause cramping and diarrhea.

On the other hand, the *body* can upset the *mind*. *Body* pain can reciprocally affect the brain's pain reception, mood, and behavior. Suppose you believe that you originally hurt your back while lifting. You can experience fear and anxiety—even panic—if you believe that you have a bad back and are called upon to lift something again, even something light. These emotions can actually increase your distress not only by making it more likely that the pain will occur, but also that the pain will be more intense.

Mind over matter

Research now shows that production of these neuropeptides in the *mind* can be turned on and off through thought, belief, relaxation, exercise, diet, sleep, and medication (Figure 4.5). Furthermore, perceptions, emotions, and attitudes exist not only in the *mind* but also in the physiology of the *body*. An individual can, through attitude and action, regulate the biochemistry and physiology of the *mind* and *body*.

Another person or other people can influence your physiology if their attitudes and actions affect your mental state. This is additional evidence of the *mind-body-spirit* connection and the interconnectedness of all living beings.

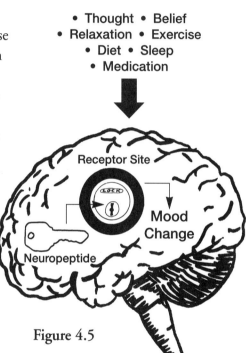

Figure 4.5

A Fourth System?

It may be that the meridian system of acupuncture represents a fourth *mind-body-spirit* communication system. This system mediates *mind-body-spirit* relations according to ancient Oriental theory and health practice. In Chapter 39, you will learn that acupuncture has been approved by the Food and Drug Administration for certain indications (e.g., nausea and vomiting of pregnancy). Research with acupuncture is proceeding at several medical centers in the United States.

"Abnormal" Pain Processing and Sensitivity in the Mind (Brain)

The *mind-body-spirit* connection does not function well in the transmission and regulation of the flow of information from the *mind* to the *body* and back in people who have fibromyalgia and other functional symptoms and syndromes. The main problem seems to be "abnormal" pain processing and sensitivity in the *mind* (Figure 4.6).
In the next chapter, you will discover that this can be explained by an abnormal central stress response in the *mind*.

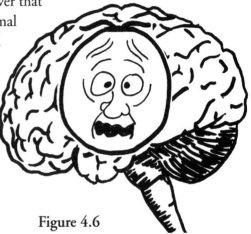

While most of the scientific evidence indicates that this processing problem and sensitivity is located in the *mind,* there is some evidence that at least part of the sensitivity problem is located in certain parts of the *body.* For example, in fibromyalgia, there is some evidence that the muscles are sensitive.

Figure 4.6

Gate-Control Theory

The *mind* can modify the feeling (perception) of *body* pain and symptoms. Signals coming from the *body* and musculoskeletal system to the *mind* through the spinal cord can be either enhanced (worsened) or blocked (lessened or stopped) through what doctors call the "descending inhibitory pathway." This important concept is illustrated in Figure 4.7.

For example, concentrating on and thinking about something else—like working hard, playing a sport, or watching a movie—can "close the gate" to the sensation of pain by the brain by sending a blocking message down the inhibitory pathway. Stress reduction techniques (Chapter 21), cognitive behavioral therapies (Chapter 22), and some medications like antidepressant drugs (Chapter 23) can also close the gate and relieve pain.

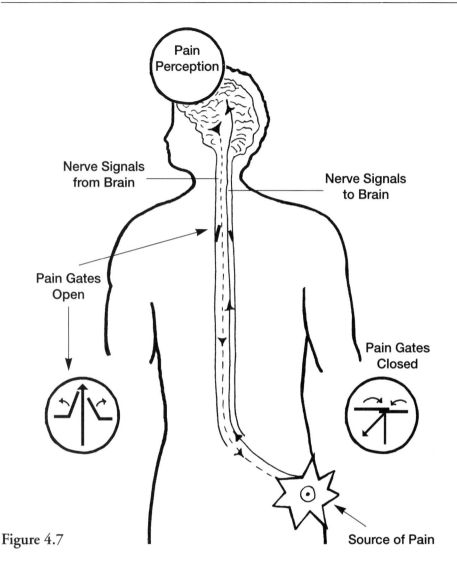

Figure 4.7

By contrast, stress, emotional distress (like anxiety or depression), and memory (like that of mental, physical, or sexual abuse) can "open the gate" to reception of pain by impeding the blocking message. This increases the perception and sensation of uncomfortable symptoms like the pain and stiffness of fibromyalgia in the *mind*.

You will explore the important role of stress, emotional distress, and memory in the *mind-body-spirit* connection in the next three chapters.

Chapter 5

Stress

(Definition of stress): In medicine, a physical, chemical, or emotional development that causes strains that can lead to physical illness.
– Microsoft® Encarta® Encyclopedia

The mind is its own place, and in itself can make a heaven of hell, a hell of heaven.
– *Paradise Lost* (1667)
John Milton

What is food to one is to others bitter poison.
– Lucretius (Titus Lucretius Carus)

You know the feeling: you have a close call in your car. Your heart races, you feel short of breath, and a slight sweat breaks out. This is an example of the "fight-or-flight" response. Stress is embodied.

Stress Defined

Margaret A. Caudill, M.D., Ph.D., author of *Managing Pain Before It Manages You* (Boston: The Guilford Press, 1995) defines stress as "the perception of a physical or psychological threat and the perception of being ill-prepared to cope with the threat." Such negative stress can be associated with both emotional and physical symptoms.

Stressors, Perception, and the Stress Response

Potentially harmful external forces, like extreme weather or the trauma of an accident or surgery, are examples of external stress and are called "stressors." But, stress also describes what happens internally (inside the *mind* and *body*) in response to external processes that are considered, or perceived, to be threatening. The emotional and chemical reaction elicited inside the *mind* and *body* is called "the stress response." Perception is why stress is personal and unique for everyone. For example, many experience a stress response when called upon to speak in public; others do not.

"Fight-or-Flight" Stress Response—What Happens When You Are Confronted by a Saber-toothed Tiger

The fight-or-flight stress response is the reaction of the *mind* and *body* to perceived stress, which is mediated through the *mind-body-spirit* connection. Adrenaline, cortisol, and growth hormone are released. Your *mind* and *body* prepare for what seems to be an emergency: your blood pressure, breathing, heart rate, metabolism, and brain activity all increase. Blood flow to the skin and internal organs decreases, but it increases to the muscles of the arms and legs. Muscle tension increases in order to prepare you to be able to fight or flee. Digestive symptoms like cramping and diarrhea can also occur.

This fight-or-flight reaction is built into your physiology and is difficult to control. It was originally designed as a survival mechanism for our primitive ancestors who were often confronted with very real and life-threatening dangers. Had you been there, you would have needed the fight-or-flight response to escape from the saber-toothed tiger that suddenly appeared out of the bush!

The "Tiger in the Mind"

For most people, life-threatening encounters are rare, but the saber-toothed tiger is always in *mind*. The "tiger in the *mind*" is the day-to-day worries and strain that keep the *mind* in a constant state of fear, anxiety, and depression and the *body* in a constant state of activation and tension. Most of the stresses that you face daily are actually false alarms; however, you cannot usually physically flee and burn the energy and tension called forth in the fight-or-flight response. Instead, you suffer the consequences as the stress response keeps recurring. As you will learn in the next chapter, a fear response in the context of stress is not necessarily a conscious experience. It is only when the emotion becomes conscious that a feeling of anxiety is experienced. Repeated fight-or-flight response is harmful stress.

Over the long haul, during perpetual or repeated stress, the *body* can be strained beyond its capability to restore balance and the normal state. Neuropeptides that are released by the brain as the *mind* responds to perceived stress (conscious and unconscious) appear to depress the immune system, which is our natural defense against infection and cancer. Furthermore, this stress response can contribute to or aggravate an existing disease or produce functional symptoms and syndromes.

Many physical symptoms and problems can occur as a consequence of harmful stress: muscular pain (including fibromyalgia and myofascial pain), fatigue, sleeplessness, functional gastrointestinal symptoms (like irritable bowel syndrome), headache, high blood pressure,

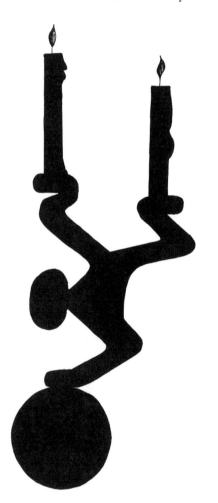

Stress by Shelley Salt

heart disease, and a generally lowered pain threshold. This physical reaction to stress can also contribute to psychological symptoms, such as increased anxiety, depression, anger, and hostility.

Lack of Margin

You didn't sleep well last night, and you're late for work. There is no time for breakfast. You always get diarrhea in the morning before going to work, especially when you have to hurry. This morning you don't even feel that you have time to go to the bathroom because you will be just that much later for work. You have a big project to complete and the deadline is this week. Morning headaches are common. You always seem to be late. It seems that you are flying from one task to the next, with no time to think, let alone relax. You really need to be in three places at the same time. You have no margin!

Richard A. Swenson, M.D., an Associate Clinical Professor in the Department of Family Medicine at the University of Wisconsin Medical School, talks about "margin" in his book, *Margin: Restoring Emotional, Physical, Financial, and Time Reserves to Overloaded Lives* (Colorado Springs, Colorado: NavPress, 1992). "Margin is the amount allowed beyond that which is needed. It is something held in reserve for contingencies or unanticipated situations. Margin is the gap between rest and exhaustion, the space between breathing freely and suffocating. It is the leeway we once had between ourselves and our limits." Dr. Swenson emphasizes that margin is the opposite of overload, and that there is no margin if overload is present.

We physicians see many marginless people every day who are exhausted, overloaded, and chronically stressed. Patients come to us with functional *mind-body-spirit* symptoms, emotional distress, and illness like fibromyalgia that cannot be explained by tests. Lack of margin is a stress that is related to these symptoms, emotional distress, and illness.

Chemical Pain Mediators and Fibromyalgia

Fibromyalgia is fundamentally related to an abnormal stress response operating primarily at the *mind* (brain) level. Evidence is accumulating that fibromyalgia is an illness associated with widespread pain sensitivity. The threshold for pain is reduced. Furthermore, pain and symptoms may be generated by stimuli that would not ordinarily be provocative. Doctors call this allodynia.

Several neuropeptide chemical messengers mediate this hypersensitivity. Many of these have been identified and implicated by Jon Russell, M.D., Ph.D., and colleagues at the University of Texas Health Sciences Center at San Antonio. These include such chemical transmitters as nerve growth factor, serotonin, dynorphin A, and substance P. As Dr. Russell,

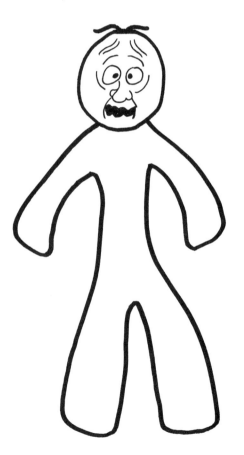

a rheumatologist and specialist in fibromyalgia, stated at the 1998 annual meeting of the American Pain Society in San Diego, "I can't say we understand this yet, but we now know there is really something wrong (biochemically)."

Jack Waxman, M.D., rheumatologist at both the Ochsner Clinic and Tulane University in New Orleans, stated that he believes the neurochemical influences on fibromyalgia often are secondary to an abnormal response to stress, which he calls "the driving force" behind the illness in most patients. He said, "Certainly, more than two-thirds of patients say it started out with some kind of traumatic event, be it physical or emotional, that caused sleep loss and great stress." He added that some hormonal stressors, like early menopause, might be sufficient to induce a fibromyalgia response.

Drugs are being developed to interfere with pain sensitivity in fibromyalgia and other related functional symptoms and syndromes, such as irritable bowel syndrome. But Dr. Waxman further stated, "My prediction is that they may help, but until you stop the central drive, you will not be dealing with the major influences on the illness for most of the patients."

We would "stress" that the symptoms of fibromyalgia are real and not imagined and that they are indeed related to neurochemical transmitters as has been discussed in Chapter 4 and in this chapter. But it is the *mind-body-spirit* connection that provides all of us—people, patients, and doctors—with a way to understand fibromyalgia. *Mind* cannot be separated from *body* and *spirit*. Illness and disease cannot be thought of as either *mind* (stress/emotion/memory) or *body* (chemical/physical).

What Is Food to One Is to Others Bitter Poison

The way you cope with stressful events may be as important as the stressors themselves relative to influencing health or illness. Stanford's Kenneth Pelletier, Ph.D., writes, "A variety of psychological factors—including mood, personality characteristics, coping style, suppressed anger, a sense of hopelessness, psychological vulnerability, and defensiveness—can all affect the way a person deals with stress and thus can potentially modulate the impact that stress will have on the immune system" (*Mind Body Medicine,* New York: Consumer Reports Books, 1993, edited by Goleman and Gurin).

Conscious and Unconscious Mind

The importance of stress management will be addressed in Chapter 21, but first understand that you have both a conscious and an unconscious *mind.* Stress in the conscious *mind* is perceived; you are aware of it. Here you can sense that you are under stress with overwork, sleep deprivation, or by your relationship with others. But stress can affect you at an unconscious level of *mind* as well, and you are not aware of this type of stress effect.

Both conscious and unconscious *mind* are particularly important relative to emotion and memory and play important roles in the perception and even generation of functional symptoms and syndromes through the *mind-body-spirit* connection.

You will learn about emotional distress and mind in the next chapter.

Chapter 6
Emotional Distress and Mind

Brain chemistry does not initiate dysfunction . . . chemistry is in the service of the psyche. In the mindbody process the physicochemical machine is driven by the emotions, not vice versa. The word psyche, derived from the Greek, means "soul."
— *The Mindbody Prescription*
John Sarno, M.D.

By understanding how fear and other negative emotions adversely affect healing, you may more easily identify how you are interfering, consciously or unconsciously, with your own healing process.
— *Why People Don't Heal, and How They Can*
Carolyn Myss, Ph.D.

In short, I learned that it is not unscientific to talk about a biology of hope—or of any of the positive emotions.
— *Head First: The Biology of Hope*
Norman Cousins

There are many different locations within the *mind* (brain) that are involved with *body* sensation and feeling, and all are connected. One of these areas relates to location and intensity of pain, and another very important area is concerned with memory and emotion. It is through the *mind-body-spirit* connection that perceived stress, emotion, memory, thoughts, and life experiences affect our perception and feeling of pain and symptoms. Emotions are embodied.

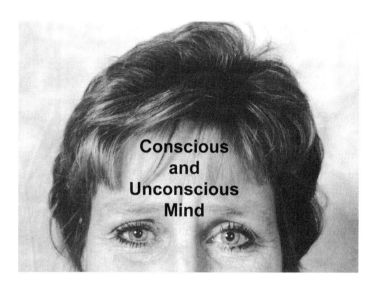

Conscious Mind

You are aware of emotion that resides within your conscious *mind.* Emotions here include anxiety, depression, anger, and fear. You *perceive* these emotions; that is, you are aware of them. These emotions of which you are aware may actually be symptoms, just like the pain of fibromyalgia and of irritable bowel syndrome. Research on the relationship of pain and emotion has concentrated on perceived emotions. These are not repressed into the unconscious brain.

Studies with functional gastrointestinal disorders (gastrointestinal *mind-body-spirit* symptoms and syndromes) confirm that conscious psychological symptoms and problems like depression and anxiety are not the cause of the symptoms. Here is why. Research shows that 15 to 20 percent of the U.S. population have the symptoms of irritable bowel syndrome (IBS). Psychological tests on these people with symptoms of irritable bowel syndrome show no differences on average than tests done on people who do not have symptoms of irritable bowel syndrome. However, when people with the symptoms of irritable bowel syndrome consult with a doctor, they become patients diagnosed with a functional syndrome called irritable bowel syndrome. These patients who have irritable bowel syndrome are found to be considerably more likely to have psychological symptoms or problems if psychological testing is conducted. These observations appear to be true for fibromyalgia as well.

There are three important implications here regarding conscious emotional distress and psychological problems.

1. Perceived emotional problems are not necessarily the cause of functional symptoms and syndromes.
2. They do affect the illness experience. It is as if these emotions amplify the experiencing of the symptoms, increase the likelihood that people will consider themselves to be ill with them, and also increase the likelihood that they will seek consultation with a doctor about them.
3. It is important for patients and for doctors to recognize and diagnose conscious emotional problems like anxiety and depression. Treatment can result in symptom relief, both emotional and physical (see Step 4).

Unconscious Mind

There is an unconscious *mind* where emotional distress is not perceived. For example, most patients who are depressed do not come in for the consultation and announce, "Doctor, I've come to see you because I have a depressed mood and take no pleasure in anything anymore." Instead, they describe their illness through functional symptoms like headache, fatigue, musculoskeletal pain, and abdominal discomfort, without necessarily being aware that they are depressed. There are reasons for this, including the fact that people may be embarrassed or feel stigmatized by a psychiatric diagnosis.

Furthermore, there is evidence that unconscious emotion may be a key to understanding functional symptoms and syndromes and how they can be treated. Dr. John Sarno, Professor of Clinical Rehabilitation Medicine at New York University School of Medicine, has identified a primary role for emotions within the unconscious *mind* in the causation of functional symptoms, such as the pain and fatigue of fibromyalgia. He calls them *mindbody* symptoms. He presents his research and experience in his book,

The Mindbody Prescription: Healing the Body, Healing the Pain, (New York: Warner Books, 1998).

Dr. Sarno proposes that it is emotion within the unconscious *mind,* mainly anger and rage, which is intolerable to the conscious *mind* and is, therefore, repressed. This pressure and rage in the unconscious *mind* derives from experiences in infancy and childhood, self-imposed pressure, and the reaction to the stresses of everyday life. As these undesirable feelings struggle to be acknowledged, the conscious *mind* prevents them from emerging into consciousness by creating what he calls, *mindbody* symptoms—such as the pain and fatigue of fibromyalgia—as a diversion. In psychological language, this is the same thing as a "defense mechanism." In other words, *mind-body-spirit* symptoms are designed by the *mind* to focus attention on the *body* and to prevent dangerous, unpleasant, and unbearable emotions in the unconscious mind from escaping into the conscious mind. Dr. Sarno further believes, as do we, that everyone harbors repressed anger and rage and that it is normal. This is why *mind-body-spirit* symptoms are so common.

Dr. Sarno describes this striving of powerful unconscious emotion into consciousness as "the drive to consciousness." Yale philosopher and psychoanalyst Jonathan Lear calls it "yearning for expression" and a desire for "conscious unification of thought and feeling" (*Love and Its Place in Nature: A Philosophical Interpretation of Freudian Psychoanalysis,* New York: Evans, 1990). Freud wrote in *Beyond the Pleasure Principle,* "The unconscious mind has no other endeavor than to break through the pressure weighing down on it and force its way either to consciousness or to a discharge through some real action."

This concept—the idea that the purpose of symptoms, physical *(body)* or emotional *(mind),* is to prevent repressed feelings from becoming consciously perceived by diversion—is a difficult one to confirm through research. Psychometric testing tools identify conscious, but not unconscious, emotion.

The practical implication of Dr. Sarno's proposal is that it is not necessary to uncover and identify the unconscious emotion. This is fortunate because accessing unconscious emotion requires analytical psychotherapy, which is time-consuming, expensive, and increasingly hard to come by in the managed-care health environment. Symptom relief comes through realizing that everyone experiences *mind-body-spirit* symptoms related to unconscious emotion. Healing comes by recognizing and accepting that the *mind* is using the *body* as a diversion.

Emotion within Our Worlds (Fields)

Rabbi Edwin H. Friedman pioneered the application of systemic concepts to families and organizations in his book, *Generation to Generation* (New York: The Guilford Press, 1985). He emphasized that it is the nature of, and our position within, the "emotional fields" of our families, relationships, communities, organizations, and work that significantly determine our individual function and symptoms. Everyone has a range of function, including potential to experience *symptoms,* and this range is influenced by these emotional fields and one's position within them. It is by becoming aware of the nature of these fields and the position within them that one can experience symptom relief. In order to do this, everyone needs to develop what he calls "self-differentiation," or strong self.

Memory

As you learned in Chapter 2, memory is important. Powerful memories can exist in both the conscious and unconscious *mind.* Real *body* symptoms can occur in association with memory. If you did not do so while reading Chapter 2, try to recall a conscious memory associated with powerful stress and/or emotion. Remember one of the most stressful or embarrassing experiences of your life. Can you feel now how your *body* felt then?

Painful memories

In the next chapter, you will learn more about the effects of memory on *mind* and *body.*

Chapter 7
Memory of Abuse

Darkness revealed is the beginning of suffering healed.
– Abused Beyond Words
Moriah S. St.Clair

You are never alone.
– The Legend of Bagger Vance
Stephen Pressfield

> The significance of memory relative to functional *mind-body-spirit* symptoms and syndromes is evident in a history of abuse. Memory is embodied.

Research

Douglas A. Drossman, M.D., is a gastroenterologist from the University of North Carolina who is a world authority on functional gastrointestinal disorders such as irritable bowel syndrome. He has emphasized that there is a new awareness and attention in the lay media and medical community about the frequency and significance of sexual, physical, and emotional abuse in America ("Sexual and physical abuse and gastrointestinal illness." *Ann Intern Med.* 1995;123:782–794). It is now clear that many people have unwanted sexual or physical abuse experiences as children or adults. Some of these occur with playmates or friends and some with family members or relatives. These experiences can be so upsetting that they may never have been discussed with anyone. They can be forgotten for long periods of time or they can come to mind frequently.

40

Mind Consequences

Psychiatrists and psychologists now recognize some emotional and psychiatric problems that can result from abuse. These include somatization and somatoform disorder, severe depression, post-traumatic stress disorder, the dissociative disorders, borderline personality disorder, and multiple personality disorder.

Body Consequences

Recent research has shown the importance of a history of physical, emotional, and sexual abuse in fibromyalgia, irritable bowel syndrome, and other functional symptoms and syndromes. There is now strong evidence that many patients with chronic functional digestive tract disorders like irritable bowel syndrome have a history of abuse, particularly if the symptoms are severe and have not responded to the usual treatments. Studies also show that people with these unpleasant and traumatic experiences see doctors more often than do those who have not been traumatized.

Two recent studies published in the medical journal called *Arthritis and Rheumatism* concluded that sexual abuse was associated with more severe symptoms of fibromyalgia but did not appear to be the cause (*Arthritis and Rheumatism,* 38:229–234 and 38:235–241).

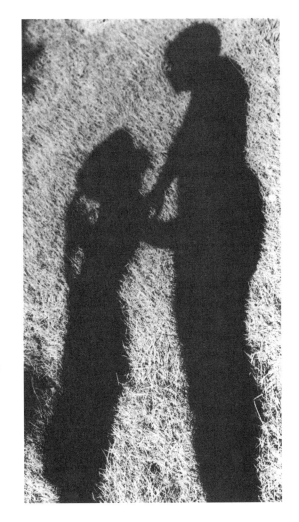

Therefore, the conscious and/or unconscious memory and stress of physical, sexual, or emotional abuse can contribute to persistent pain, resistance to treatment, and frequent doctor visits.

Implications for Treatment

Doctors have only recently begun to understand how common a history of abuse is in patients who suffer from *mind-body-spirit* syndromes like fibromyalgia. Studies show that most patients do not volunteer this information, so doctors need to be on the lookout for this history, particularly when the symptoms are severe or chronic, unexplained, and unresponsive to treatment. If the doctor knows of this history, then he or she can better understand the illness or condition, which may lead to improvement through psychological treatment.

If you have a history of abuse, whether it is mental, physical, or sexual, it is important that you share the information with a trusted caregiver. Failure to recognize the relationship of strong memories and *mind-body-spirit* symptoms and syndromes can interfere with your healing.

In the next chapter, we will explain why we are introducing new terms in this book relative to the *mind-body-spirit* connection.

Chapter 8

A New and Shared Language for People, Patients, and Doctors

I hope I have convinced you of some simple but far-reaching
truths. That our mental state and physical health are inexorably
intertwined. . . . That the relationship between mind and health
is mediated by both our behavior and by biological connections
between the brain and the immune system. That these connections
work in both directions, so our physical health can influence our
mental state. That all illnesses have psychological and emotional
consequences as well as causes.

– *The Healing Mind*
Paul Martin, Ph.D.

Fibromyalgia is "cured" by teaching people to be aware
of the nature of the mindbody connection.

– *The Mindbody Prescription*
John Sarno, M.D.

A remarkable fact is that most of the common *body* symptoms that
cause people to see doctors cannot be explained by medical science.
Unfortunately, this makes both patients and doctors very unhappy.

What We Have Here Is a Failure to Communicate

Earlier in this book, you learned that most of the symptoms that bring
people to doctors are called "functional" because they cannot be explained
by test results (see Table 2 in the introduction, *Your Prescription for
Change!*). So people with functional symptoms become patients when

they consult with doctors who diagnose functional syndromes, which are collections of functional symptoms (see Chapter 17).

You may know from experience how frustrating it is as a patient to have real and distressing symptoms, only to be told that the tests are normal. Furthermore, it is likely that you left the doctor's office without knowing why you hurt and what you could do about the pain. As doctors, we can tell you how frustrating it is for us to seemingly be unable to be of more help. Take a look at this problem from the perspectives of both patients and doctors, and consider the patient-doctor relationship.

Patients' perspective

Most people and patients do not understand the *mind-body-spirit* connection. Furthermore, terms like "functional," "psychosomatic," and "somatization" are often understood by patients to mean that doctors

- Do not believe that the symptoms are real
- Attribute the *body* symptoms purely to "stress"
- Suspect that a mental illness or serious psychological problem must be present
- May be missing a serious disease that has not yet been identified
- Should be able to treat and cure the symptoms because a precise medical diagnosis of a syndrome has been made

The doctors' perspective

In a perfect world, doctors would utilize a biopsychosocialspiritual approach to the diagnosis and treatment of illness and disease. However, in the real world, some doctors do not accept this model. Very few doctors use the language of the *mind-body-spirit* connection with patients. If they do, it is very difficult to apply the biopsychosocialspiritual/*mind-body-spirit* approach in the managed care environment with rushed encounters and declining reimbursements for time spent talking with patients.

The patient-doctor relationship

You will learn about healing and the importance of the patient-doctor relationship in Step 3. Stan Sateren, M.D., has said, "The *spirit* of dialog provides opportunities for healing," (*Irritable Bowel Syndrome & the Mind-Body/Brain-Gut Connection,* by William B. Salt II, M.D., Columbus: Parkview Publishing, 1997).

Unfortunately, many patients and doctors either do not understand or do not accept the *mind-body-spirit* connection. Both groups may underestimate the power of knowledge and patients' ability to heal. The "failure to communicate" translates into frustrated and unhappy patients and doctors. Dr. Edward Shorter, a professor of medical history at the University of Toronto has written, "With each passing year, the gap between doctor and patient widens, as doctors retreat increasingly into a shell of resentment and patients become ever more exasperated with the impersonality of care." (*Doctors and Their Patients: A Social History,* New Jersey: Transaction Publishers, 1991).

A New and Shared Language

We are convinced that people with symptoms, patients with syndromes, and doctors who diagnose them need to accept and understand the biopsychosocialspiritual/*mind-body-spirit* connection and that a new and shared language is needed (Figure 8.1). We propose the following new terms:

MindBodySpirit Connection
MindBodySpirit Symptoms
MindBodySpirit Syndromes
MindBodySpirit Healing

The MindBodySpirit Connection

The *mind* and *body* are linked. Even though symptoms are not "all in the head," the organ in the head—the brain *(mind)*—is linked to the *body.* Communication is a two-way street via the spinal cord. Furthermore, the *mind* and *body* communicate through neurochemical pathways that are even capable of transmitting emotion (Chapter 4). Finally, stress, emotional distress, thoughts, and memory, including that within the unconscious brain, all play important roles relative to symptoms (Chapters 5–7).

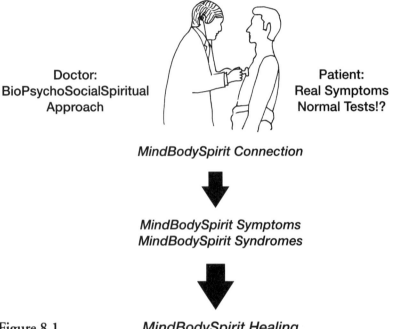

**Understanding Functional Bodily
Symptoms and Syndromes:
A New and Shared Language**

Doctor:
BioPsychoSocialSpiritual
Approach

Patient:
Real Symptoms
Normal Tests!?

MindBodySpirit Connection

MindBodySpirit Symptoms
MindBodySpirit Syndromes

Figure 8.1   *MindBodySpirit Healing*

Dr. Candace Pert has recommended that the term *mind-body* should no longer be hyphenated. Dr. John Sarno endorses this, and we agree. But we include *spirit* to yield the new term *MindBodySpirit Connection*.

MindBodySpirit Symptoms

We recommend that symptoms formerly termed functional, psychosomatic, or somatization now be collectively called *MindBodySpirit Symptoms*.

MindBodySpirit Syndromes

We propose that functional syndromes, such as fibromyalgia and irritable bowel syndrome, be called *MindBodySpirit Syndromes*.

MindBodySpirit Healing

Finally, we call for people with symptoms, patients with syndromes, and doctors who diagnose them to "see" a new way of addressing illness and disease, especially *MindBodySpirit Symptoms* and *MindBodySpirit Syndromes*. This *MindBodySpirit Healing* practiced by doctors and caregivers to promote health and healing includes the best of biomedicine with the biopsychosocialspiritual approach.

Doctors, people, and patients underestimate each individual's power to heal. *MindBodySpirit Healing* is based upon recognition, understanding, and acceptance of several important concepts.

- The *MindBodySpirit Connection*
- The difference between disease and illness and between treatment and healing
- The *body's* innate healing potential
- The patient's acceptance of responsibility in healing
- The healing power of the patient-doctor relationship

Methods of *MindBodySpirit Healing* include combinations of the following:

- Diet (Chapter 26)
- Exercise (Chapters 29 and 30)
- Cognitive behavioral therapy: learning how to change thoughts, perceptions, and behaviors to control symptoms (Chapter 22)
- Relaxation therapy and stress management, such as breathing techniques and meditation (Chapter 21)
- Medication (like antidepressant drugs) which can either help treat any psychological dimension (such as anxiety or depression) or act as pain relievers by stimulating the brain to send signals which block transmission of pain to the brain (Chapter 23)
- Prayer (Chapter 3)
- Alternative and complementary therapy (Chapters 39 and 40)

Why a New Language?

We believe that this language is shared, inclusive, integrated, holistic, contemporary, positive, and connecting.

- **Shared**   A common language improves everyone's chances to communicate effectively and be understood. Most importantly, it reduces medical "jargon" that patients have a difficult time with, particularly when they have real symptoms and tests are found to be normal.

- **Inclusive**   *Spirit* is included with *mind* and *body* because of increasing evidence of the intersection of the mystifying power of *spirit* and healing (Chapter 3).

- **Integrated**   Removing the hyphens more directly represents the *MindBodySpirit Connection* in a visual and symbolic way.

- **Holistic**   The *mind, body,* and *spirit* are connected. It no longer makes sense to classify symptoms as either *mind* (stress/emotion/thought/memory), *body* (chemical/physical) or *spirit* (soul related).

- **Modern**   The biomedical model of health and illness prevails, but you have seen the superiority of the biopsychosocialspiritual model (Chapter 2). The *MindBodySpirit Connection* can serve as professional language for this model while being more easily understood by the public.

- **Positive**   Words like "functional," "psychosomatic," and "somatization" have assumed a negative connotation. These symptoms and syndromes are real and neither imagined nor phoney. New language removes any stigmatization and permits all of us to start anew. *MindBodySpirit* is an uplifting, validating, hopeful way of describing.

- **Connecting**   We believe that this contemporary and inclusive terminology and language will help everyone—people, patients, and doctors—to communicate with one another about these very real symptoms and syndromes. Everyone needs to understand the nature and power of the *MindBodySpirit Connection.* We want to see patients and doctors use this language with one another. With these terms, people and patients can better understand these symptoms and syndromes and their power to heal; doctors can appreciate their power to treat and assist their patients; and patients and doctors can speak the same language in order to achieve a common purpose: healing.

In the next step, you will learn what you need to know about your *MindBodySpirit Syndrome:* fibromyalgia. It will be your second step to healing.

REVIEW OF STEP 1

1. Most people experience unwanted *body* symptoms that cannot be explained by tests. Doctors diagnose these symptoms as functional, psychosomatic, or somatization symptoms.

2. It is important to understand the difference between disease and illness as well as the difference between treatment and healing. These differences are best appreciated through the biopsychosocialspiritual model of health, disease, and illness.

3. The *mind* and *body* are inextricably linked and communicate via a two-way pathway via the spinal cord. Furthermore, chemicals called neuropeptides transmit information, including emotional information, throughout the body.

4. Because *spirit* is important in healing, we propose the more appropriate term *MindBodySpirit Connection.*

5. Repeated "fight-or-flight" response produces harmful stress. The *body* can be strained beyond its capability to restore balance, resulting in physical symptoms. Beware of the tiger in the mind.

6. It is through the *MindBodySpirit Connection* that conscious and unconscious perceived stress, emotional distress—like anxiety, depression, and anger—and memory affect and influence whether and to what extent and degree we experience functional symptoms, whether we feel ill or unwell with them, whether we will miss work or social opportunities, and whether we will report them to doctors. Healing begins by understanding and accepting this.

7. Many people with fibromyalgia also have other unexplained symptoms where tests are normal—the most common of which are insomnia/difficulty sleeping and fatigue. These symptoms represent illness without disease and are what doctors call "functional," "psychosomatic," or "somatization" symptoms. We propose that these symptoms be called *MindBodySpirit Symptoms.*

8. Fibromyalgia is a *MindBodySpirit Symptom* complex, with widespread musculoskeletal pain, fatigue, and sleep disturbance. It is what we call a *MindBodySpirit Syndrome.*

9. We are proposing a new and shared language to help people with symptoms, patients with syndromes, and doctors who diagnose them to communicate about symptoms and syndromes in order to achieve a common purpose: healing.

STEP 2

LEARNING ABOUT FIBROMYALGIA AND MYOFASCIAL PAIN

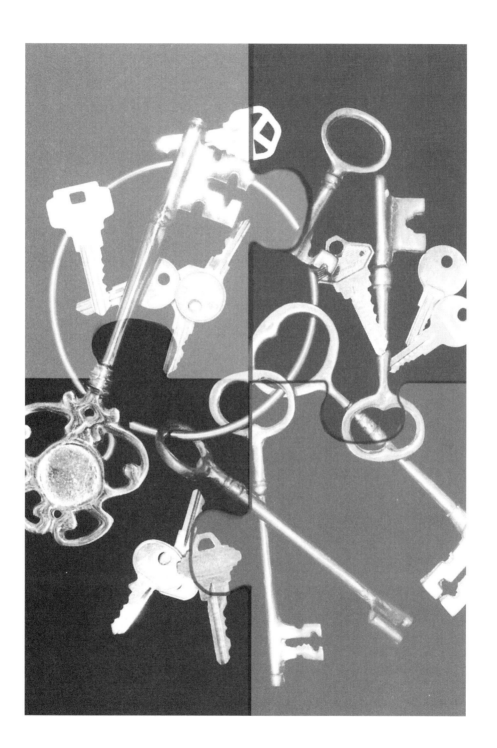

Chapter 9
Definition of Fibromyalgia

Our body is precious. It is a vehicle for awakening. Treat it with care.
– Buddha

Many people with the symptoms of widespread *body* pain and fatigue are diagnosed with a syndrome called *fibromyalgia.* Disability from pain and fibromyalgia is increasing every year in American industry.

Definition of Fibromyalgia

Fibromyalgia, a *MindBodySpirit Syndrome,* affects mostly women. It is a form of nonarticular (nonjoint) rheumatism (pain) that is characterized by both widespread muscular aching and stiffness as well as by tenderness upon palpation (pressing the finger or thumb) of specified sites called trigger or tender points. These trigger points are mainly located in the neck, back, and extremities. Trigger points will be discussed in more detail in Chapter 16.

Most with fibromyalgia have two other *MindBodySpirit Symptoms:*

- Fatigue
- Sleep disturbance (Chapter 25)

Furthermore, in Chapter 8 you learned that many with fibromyalgia have other "functional" *MindBodySpirit Symptoms* and *MindBodySpirit Syndromes,* including

- Tension headaches
- Irritable bowel syndrome
- Back pain

- Irritable bladder
- Chronic pelvic pain

You will learn more about these symptoms and syndromes in Chapter 17.

Tests Are Normal

With the exception of trigger (tender) points and dermatographia on physical examination (Chapter 16), tests that may be ordered are normal. Tests that might be recommended include blood studies, x-rays, CT scan, MRI, and EMG.

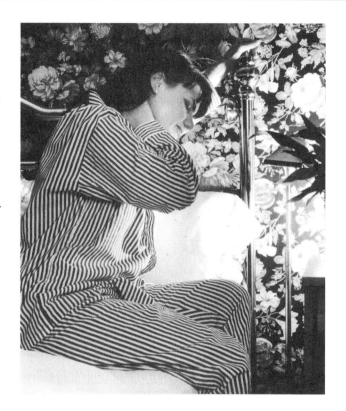

An Abnormal Test Does Not Explain Fibromyalgia

If structural findings like arthritis are found, say on an x-ray, they are most likely unrelated to any causation of fibromyalgia. This is important because many people with arthritis also have fibromyalgia and can benefit from proper diagnosis and treatment directed to fibromyalgia. Furthermore, it is important to avoid falsely attributing the symptoms of fibromyalgia to a finding on testing because to do so can interfere with healing (Chapter 12).

Symptoms

The location of the pain in fibromyalgia is described in Table 9.1.

Table 9.1		
Location of Pain in Fibromyalgia		
Base of skull	Chest	Legs
Neck	Back	Buttocks
Shoulders	Arms	Hips

Most people with fibromyalgia have intermittent symptoms that they describe as mild to moderate. Some people have painful, distressing, and disabling symptoms and go to see the doctor frequently. A few are burdened by chronic stress and/or emotional problems like anxiety and depression that actually make their symptoms worse and reduce their ability to cope. These patients can undergo expensive, unnecessary—and sometimes risky—tests, treatments, and even surgery in an effort to get the answer to their problem.

History of Fibromyalgia

Sir William Gowers first described fibromyalgia in 1904. Other terms have been used throughout the years: fibrositis, fibromyositis, myofibrositis, myofascial pain, muscular rheumatism, tension myalgia, myalgia, rheumatic myositis, and myelogelosis.

It has only been since the 1970s that physicians and scientists have studied fibromyalgia, confirmed that it is not caused by inflammation or a known disease process, and concentrated on providing medical care. Interest in this very common problem is growing, particularly since fibromyalgia is a major women's health problem and doctors now realize how widespread and distressing the problem is.

World Wide Problem, Especially for Women

Fibromyalgia has been described in most countries of the world. It does not appear to be related to ethnicity and is not a problem related to colder climates. A recent scientific study indicates that fibromyalgia affects 2 percent of people in the United States. There is a progressive increase in the prevalence with age, such that about 7 percent of women 70 years of age are affected (*Arthritis and Rheumatism.* 1995;38:19–28).

Seventy-five to ninety-five percent of the millions of Americans who suffer from fibromyalgia are women. Fibromyalgia is the most common cause of generalized musculoskeletal pain in women between the ages of 20 and 55 and is the second most common diagnosis made by rheumatologists. It is a major women's health issue and receives considerable attention by the media in newspapers, magazines, radio, and television.

In the next chapter, you will learn about *myofascial pain,* which is a localized form of fibromyalgia.

Chapter 10
Myofascial Pain Syndrome

Although passive patients may console themselves by believing
that their doctor has a magical cure for every illness, in reality
they are missing an important opportunity to contribute to
their own care and they are setting themselves up for a major
disappointment if the treatment fails.
– in *Mind Body Medicine* (edited by Goleman and Gurin)
Tom Ferguson, M.D.

Myofascial pain syndrome can be thought of simply as a type of regional or localized fibromyalgia. Myofascial pain is experienced in muscles of a given area of the body—mainly upper back, shoulders, and lower back.

Definition of Myofascial Pain Syndrome

Myofascial pain is defined by the presence of trigger points, including a localized area of deep muscle tenderness, located in a taut band in the muscle with a characteristic reference zone of perceived pain aggravated by palpation of the trigger point. Some authorities also insist on the presence of a local twitch response. This twitch response is considered to be diagnostic of an active trigger point. It is a visible or palpable contraction of the muscle that is produced by a rapid snap of the examining finger of the taut band of muscle.

Comparison of Myofascial Pain Syndrome with Fibromyalgia

Like fibromyalgia, myofascial pain syndrome occurs most often among women between the ages of 40 and 50. Fatigue, stiffness, generalized pain, and poor sleep occasionally accompany the muscle tenderness, and anxiety and depression may also be present in some individuals.

Myofascial pain syndromes may include other common local pain syndromes such as tension headaches, low back pain, cervical (neck) strain disorders, and temporomandibular joint syndrome. So, myofascial pain syndrome may be one of the most common causes of musculoskeletal pain. Table 10.1 provides a contrast and comparison of myofascial pain syndrome with fibromyalgia.

Table 10.1

Comparison of Myofascial Pain Syndrome with Fibromyalgia

Myofascial Pain Syndrome	Fibromyalgia
Local or regional pain	Diffuse pain; involves many regions
Acute or chronic onset	Gradual, insidious onset
Nonmusculoskeletal symptoms occasionally	Nonmusculoskeletal symptoms (fatigue, poor sleep, depression) are common
Trigger points localized and regionalized	Trigger points widespread and numerous (> 11)
Response to local therapy: "curative"	Response to local therapy: not sustained
Mild, temporary disability	Greater, long-lasting disability
More common among women	Female to male ratio is 10:1

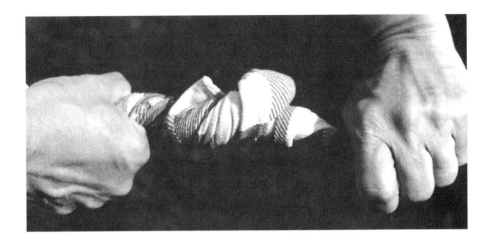

Other Regional Myofascial Pain Syndromes

Myofascial pain syndromes include other common regional pain disorders listed in Table 10.2.

Table 10.2
Other Regional Myofascial Pain Disorders
Tension headaches Low back strain Neck strain Temporomandibular joint (TMJ) syndrome Repetitive strain syndrome

Let's look at two of these, TMJ syndrome and the repetitive strain syndrome.

Temporomandibular joint (TMJ) syndrome
TMJ syndrome causes intense pain in the jaw and facial area that can radiate throughout the head and neck. Although the exact cause of TMJ syndrome is not understood, Figure 10.1 describes the factors that contribute to the syndrome.

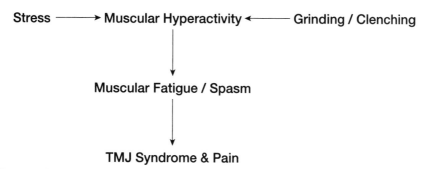

Figure 10.1

Table 10.3 lists characteristics of TMJ syndrome.

Table 10.3
Characteristics of Temporomandibular Joint (TMJ) Syndrome
• Pain localized to the jaw and facial areas • Repetitive muscle activity (grinding and clenching of the jaws and teeth) • More common between ages of 20 to 50 • Four times more common among women than men • Aggravated by stress • Associated with poor sleep • Can be helped by antidepressant drugs • Examinations and lab results usually normal

A doctor or dentist can diagnose TMJ syndrome, and much of the treatment is based upon the principles discussed throughout this book.

Repetitive strain syndrome

This term is used when myofascial pain occurs in association with activities involving repetitious movement or postural constraint. An example of repetitive strain syndrome is carpal tunnel syndrome, with pain and numbness in the hands related to continuous typing.

61

Diagnosis of Myofascial Pain Syndrome

Table 10.4 lists the clinical criteria that doctors have developed for making the diagnosis of myofascial pain syndrome.

Table 10.4

Criteria for Myofascial Pain Syndrome

A diagnosis of myofascial pain syndrome can be made if five major criteria and at least one of three minor criteria are satisfied.

Major Criteria
- Localized spontaneous pain
- Spontaneous pain or altered sensations in expected referred pain area for a given trigger point
- Taut, palpable band in accessible muscle
- Exquisite, localized tenderness in precise point along taut band
- Some measurable degree of reduced range of movement

Minor Criteria
- Reproduction of spontaneously perceived pain and altered sensations by pressure on trigger point
- Elicitation of a local twitch response of muscular fibers by transverse "snapping" palpation or by needle insertion into trigger point
- Pain relief obtained by muscle stretching or injection of trigger point

---

Adapted from Simons DG. Muscular Pain Syndromes. In Fricton JR, Awad JR, editors: *Advances in pain research and therapy.* New York: Raven Press, 1990;17:1–41

Treatment

Myofascial pain syndrome generally responds well to therapy with a good prognosis for the patient to regain full function and return to regular activities. Treatment is directed to localized symptoms. Physical therapy, spray and stretch techniques, and local injections are standard methods of treating myofascial pain.

Physical therapy may involve various treatment techniques as well as progressive exercise. Both aerobic and strength training have been proven effective for the treatment of myofascial pain syndrome (Chapters 29 and 30).

Spray and stretch is described in Chapter 32. The technique involves the application of an anesthetic spray or use of ice massage followed by firm massage or passive stretching of the painful muscle at the trigger point.

Trigger point injection is also discussed in Chapter 32. It involves injecting a local anesthetic into the tender muscle. An alternative is the reinsertion of a dry needle or injecting saline into the trigger point.

Medications are not usually effective for the long-term treatment of myofascial pain. However, mild analgesics, like acetaminophen or ibuprofen, and other nonsteroidal anti-inflammatory drugs may provide some short-term relief.

The next chapter addresses the "cause" of fibromyalgia.

Chapter 11
The "Cause" of Fibromyalgia

The Brain—is wider than the Sky—
For—put them side by side—
The one the other will contain
With ease—and You—beside—
– Emily Dickinson
(1830–1886)

The whole is greater than the sum of its parts.
– Anonymous

> Fibromyalgia is not caused by infection, inflammation, allergy, or
> an autoimmune disorder. In fact, blood tests and x-rays fail to show
> any abnormality that could account for the symptoms. But the
> symptoms are very real! What causes them?

The MindBodySpirit Connection

Before you started reading this book, perhaps you had gained the impression that your problem was "all in your head." But studies show that millions suffer from fibromyalgia, so you are clearly not alone. The symptoms are not phoney or imagined. Furthermore, your symptoms are not "all in your head." Instead, they are related to the interaction and linkage of your *mind, body,* and *spirit:* the *MindBodySpirit Connection.*

In Step 1, you learned how this connection and communication process works. The *mind* (brain) and *body* are inextricably linked and communicate via a two-way pathway via the spinal cord. Furthermore, chemicals called neuropeptides transmit information, including emotional information, throughout the *mind* and *body.* So there is a network in the *body* through the nervous system and by way of chemical transmission that permits organs (including brain/*mind*) and *body* systems to influence and affect one another. You also learned that the scientific connection of the *mind-body* is embedded within, and connected to, the mystery of the *spirit*.

As you learn about the "cause" of fibromyalgia, keep in mind that fibromyalgia is best understood as a *MindBodySpirit Syndrome,* which is a collection of *MindBodySpirit Symptoms* (see Chapters 8 and 17).

The Important Concept of System Thinking

Thinking of the *MindBodySpirit Connection* as a system is important in understanding the "cause" of fibromyalgia. System thinking emphasizes the interrelatedness of the parts. So instead of seeing parts as being isolated and unrelated, it is important to appreciate the whole. The whole is a set of parts or components that interact. Thinking systemically requires that you look at the vital and ongoing interaction of the connected parts. When you think this way, you realize that it is not possible to understand one part or element without the other. Look at Figure 11.1.

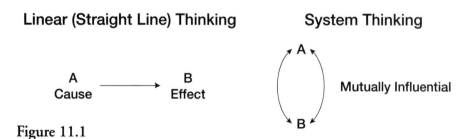

Linear (Straight Line) Thinking

A
Cause
⟶
B
Effect

System Thinking

A

B

Mutually Influential

Figure 11.1

With linear, or straight line thinking, you assume that things are influenced only in one direction; A causes B. But system thinking allows you to think in terms of loops instead of straight lines. Both A and B influence one another and each is influenced by the other.

Think of the "cause" of fibromyalgia as the consequence of interrelated components. These components are part of a system and interact with one another. No single component is the "cause" of fibromyalgia. Instead, "the whole is greater than the sum of its parts."

Figure 11.2 presents a paradigm of the "cause" of fibromyalgia from a system thinking perspective.

Mind

Some people with fibromyalgia note that its onset followed a traumatic event or experience, either physical (such as infection, accident, or injury) or emotional. Nevertheless, fibromyalgia cannot be explained by an ongoing injury or infection.

Environmental, genetic, and social factors—in conjunction with conscious and unconscious stress, emotional distress (anxiety, depression, fear, and anger), thoughts, and memory—contribute to the symptoms of fibromyalgia. Remember that chemicals called neuropeptides transmit information, including emotional information, throughout the body. The consequences include

- Abnormal pain perception and sensitivity in the *mind* (brain)
- Physiologic arousal that increases muscle tension
- Poor sleep, which contributes to fatigue and further upsets the *mind*
- Fatigue, which not only upsets the *mind*, but also leads to inactivity

Body

- The pain of fibromyalgia derives from abnormal pain perception and sensitivity, primarily at the *mind* level but possibly to some extent from increased sensitivity within the muscles themselves. Current research shows that most of this increased sensitivity and perception is operating at the *mind* (brain) level rather than the body itself.
- Muscle tension from physiologic arousal results in increased pain. A tense muscle is more pain-sensitive than a relaxed muscle.
- Inactivity and deconditioning lead to muscles that are susceptible to microinjury with activity that further enhances the pain.
- A vicious cycle is established as the pain leads to reduced activity and interferes with sleep.

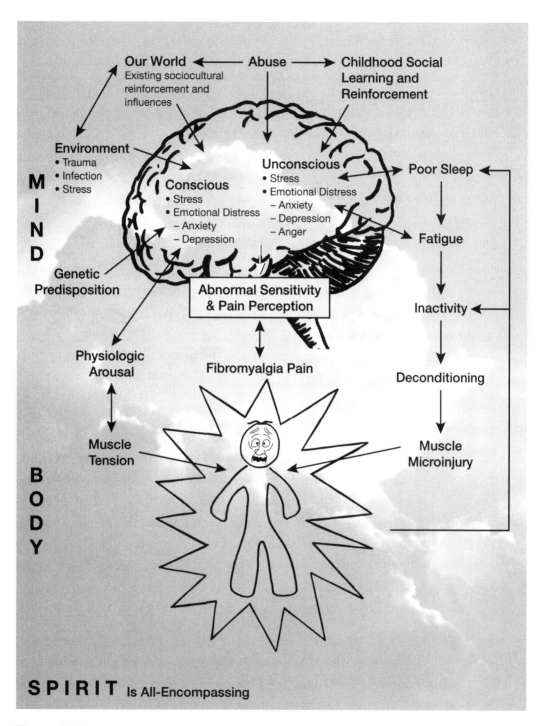

Figure 11.2

Spirit

Chapter 3 addressed the accumulating scientific evidence that spirit plays an important role in health and illness. This is why we have graphically depicted the *MindBody* within a *Spirit* cloud in Figure 11.2 to represent the *MindBodySpirit Connection.*

Modulating Factors

Some with fibromyalgia consider the following factors to aggravate their symptoms:

- **Weather**   Many find that harsh and extreme weather, such as extreme cold, damp, humid, or rainy conditions aggravate their symptoms. Some find that they feel best in the hot, dry climate of the southwestern United States.

- **Hormones (menstrual cycle)**   Women with fibromyalgia may find that their symptoms are aggravated and associated with their menstrual cycle. Fluid retention or premenstrual syndrome (PMS) can further contribute to the pain.

- **Stimulants**   Caffeine, nicotine, recreational drugs, and some medications can interfere with sleep and increase stress and anxiety. Muscle tension can be increased with the result that the pain of fibromyalgia is intensified.

- **Alcohol**   Alcohol can aggravate symptoms by interfering with sleep by its effect as a depressant. When used in excess, alcohol can have a direct and toxic effect on muscles.

- **Spontaneous "flare-ups"**   Commonly, symptoms wax and wane without apparent reason. Such "flare-ups" may seem to be unrelated to any physical, environmental, psychosocial, or emotional factor.

The *MindBodySpirit Connection* is the foundation for understanding your fibromyalgia. Healing begins with understanding, and the next step will show you how to begin the healing process based upon diagnosis and education.

REVIEW OF STEP 2

1. Fibromyalgia is defined as widespread muscular aching and stiffness associated with tenderness on palpation at specified sites called tender points.

2. Fibromyalgia is a common *MindBodySpirit Syndrome* and illness characterized by widespread musculoskeletal pain that cannot be explained by blood tests, x-rays, or other tests. But the symptoms are very real and are not "all in the head."

3. Fibromyalgia affects at least 10 million Americans and is a major women's health issue.

4. Fibromyalgia is understood through the interaction and linkage of the *mind, body,* and *spirit:* the *MindBodySpirit Connection.* Thinking of the *MindBodySpirit Connection* as a system is the key to understanding the "cause" of fibromyalgia.

5. Myofascial pain syndrome is regional fibromyalgia and is a localized area of muscular tenderness and trigger (tender) points. It includes tension headaches, low back strain, neck strain, and temporomandibular joint syndrome.

STEP 3

HEALING WITH DIAGNOSIS AND EDUCATION

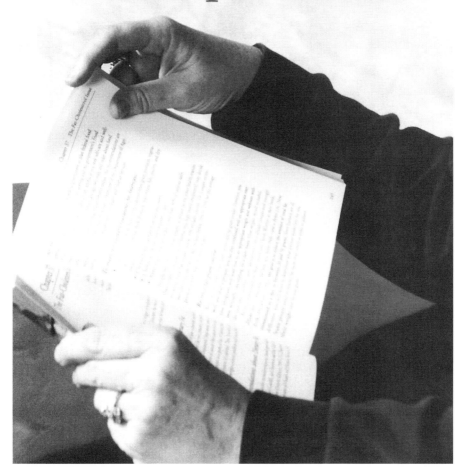

Knowledge
... powerful
... therapeutic

Chapter 12
Healing

Your mind and body are one, inextricably linked. You are
stronger than you know and have more power over your
body than you probably realize.
– *The Mindbody Prescription*
John Sarno, M.D.

Please keep in mind the distinction between healing and
treatment: treatment originates from the outside, whereas
healing comes from within.
– *8 Weeks to Optimum Health*
Andrew Weil, M.D.

> You may think that the most important step to healing is finding
> the right doctor. It's not. It is understanding *your* power to heal.

Healing Comes from Within

You have the power to heal and this comes from you. Everyone—people
with symptoms, patients with syndromes, and doctors who diagnose
them—tends to underestimate this power and potential. In the book,
Whole Healing, Elliott Dacher says, "We contain within us the wisdom
we need to be healthy," (New York: Dutton, 1996). Many physicians and
authorities are emphasizing this, including Herbert Benson, M.D.;
Deepak Chopra, M.D.; Norman Cousins; Carolyn Myss, Ph.D.; John
Sarno, M.D.; and Andrew Weil, M.D.

Distinction between Healing and Treatment

You have a natural healing system within, regardless of whether treatment is applied. Healing is internal; treatment is external. Treatments—including medications and surgery—can help make healing possible and reduce or remove factors that impede it. Nevertheless, healing and treatment are not the same and the distinction is important.

The Importance of Education

We believe that patient education is the most important part of the treatment in fibromyalgia and that for most people, it is more important than medication. As C. Everett Koop, M.D., former Surgeon General of the United States, has said, *"It's really a very simple idea: no prescription is worth more than knowledge."* Research on the best methods for providing patient education and on the beneficial effects of education is underway. We are confident of the value of education.

The MindBodySpirit Connection

You have learned how *MindBodySpirit Symptoms* like the pain and fatigue of fibromyalgia are mediated through the *MindBodySpirit Connection*. Healing comes from understanding and accepting this *"Connection."* For example, you have learned that the appreciation and acceptance of the impact of stress, emotion, and memory at the conscious and unconscious level on the *mind* and *body* can have therapeutic power in relieving *MindBodySpirit Symptoms* and *MindBodySpirit Syndromes* even if you do not perceive or fully understand the stress, emotion, thoughts, or memory.

The Healing Power of Love and Relationship

Remember that we live in relationship with others within emotional "fields," (Chapter 6). We are all "connected." Edwin Friedman has shown

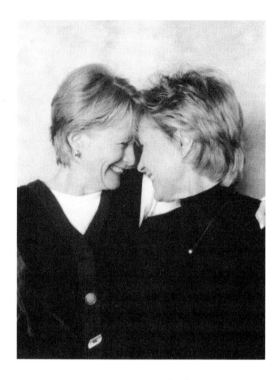

that everyone has a range of function and symptoms relative to his or her relationships with others within emotional fields.

Dr. Dean Ornish argues that loneliness is a major risk factor for heart disease in his book, *Love and Survival: The Healing Power of Intimacy* (New York: Harper-Collins, 1998). He stresses that love and companionship are as important for a healthy heart as diet and exercise. Medical evidence is accumulating that this is true for illnesses like fibromyalgia.

Social support can be defined as the number of people you have positive interactions with on a regular basis, the number and quality of friends you have, and the number of social activities and organizations in which you participate. Healthy and healing relationships can be established with God, spouse, family, friends, and even pets.

The benefit of social support and close relationships is mediated through the *MindBodySpirit Connection* by

- Reduction of the production of stress hormones (Chapter 5)
- Improvement in the ability to cope with potentially harmful emotions like depression, anxiety, and anger (Chapter 6)
- Address of painful memories (Chapter 7)
- Experience of the beneficial placebo effect (Chapters 13 and 14).
- Spirituality, faith, and relationship with a higher power (Chapter 3)

Before you learn about consulting with a doctor in Chapter 14, take a look at "the placebo effect and nocebo effect" in the next chapter.

Chapter 13
The Placebo Effect and Nocebo Effect

Among the most potent, tried and trusted remedies that rely entirely on psychology is the placebo effect—that remarkably robust phenomenon whereby we get better because we believe we are going to get better. . . . They are the twentieth century's continuation of an ancient tradition of secret potions, incantations, leeches, the royal touch, pilgrimages to healing shrines, gold tablets, and magic spells.
– *The Healing Mind*
Paul Martin, Ph.D.

There is nothing either good or bad, but thinking makes it so.
– *Hamlet* (1601)
William Shakespeare

Most of the time we think we're sick, it's all in the mind.
– *Look Homeward, Angel* (1929)
Thomas Wolfe

Belief in a treatment—even if shown to be of no value, like a sugar pill—may bring relief of symptoms. This is known as the placebo effect, but it may not bring enduring relief or cure. By contrast, negative belief can have a harmful effect.

The Placebo Effect

The word, "placebo" means "I shall please" in Latin. People taking a placebo believe it to be a real drug and experience symptom relief. This placebo effect can be remarkably powerful in treatment of such conditions as chronic pain, high blood pressure, angina, and depression. Scientific studies have confirmed that the placebo can work up to 70 percent of the time. This phenomenon is the basis for what is called the randomized double blind clinical trial in which the treatment to be tested is compared to a placebo. It is necessary to prove that the treatment is significantly better than a placebo, which can be very difficult to do. The placebo effect is very strong evidence of the *MindBodySpirit Connection!*

The placebo effect is based upon blind faith and belief. Unfortunately, relief from the symptoms is often temporary. This is the reason that many treatments for fibromyalgia like physical therapy, medication, alternative treatments, and surgery may eventually fail. The temporary benefit is related to the placebo effect. Sometimes the pain is relieved via the placebo effect through surgery only to recur later or move to another location in the body. Doctors call this "symptom shifting."

The Nocebo Effect

A nocebo is the opposite of a placebo and can cause sickness or illness from a negative effect. The word, *nocebo,* actually means "I will harm."

Belief can work against people. As an extreme example of the nocebo effect, belief in a life-threatening danger can induce excessive amounts of stress hormones that can trigger a chain of chemical events in the body, which can lead to death. The nocebo effect is one of the principles that underlies voodoo practices. The belief in voodoo can be so strong, that when cursed by the witch doctor, the believer immediately collapses and dies. There is no physical reason for death—only the *belief and fear* that the curse causes death! Voodoo is still practiced in some countries today.

Other examples of the nocebo effect, in addition to belief-engendered death, are mass psychogenic illness (such as when children in a school all develop a headache when they believe that they have been exposed to a toxic substance) and "memories" of having been abducted by aliens.

By dwelling upon worst-case scenarios, exaggerated risks, doubts, and worries, you can allow the nocebo effect to affect your *body* in harmful ways. The *body* can be persuaded to be sick when there is no biologic reason. This is illness without disease (Chapter 2).

The Nocebo Effect in Fibromyalgia

If you are informed that the pain of your fibromyalgia is related to inflammation of the muscles or that your back pain is caused by a herniated disc, then the nocebo effect can ensure that your pain will continue. If you are advised to remain inactive and not to exercise, you believe the problem to be quite serious and experience a worsening of the pain. A further consequence is deconditioning with weakening of muscles and loss of muscle tissue. This adds to the problem.

When the pain continues, tests are ordered. If the MRI or CT scan shows not only a herniated disc, but also that there is arthritis of the spine, you become convinced that you have a "bad back." Pain intensifies, especially if you are told that you may need surgery if you fail to respond to more conservative measures.

The diagnosis that is based upon a muscle disease or deficiency or upon a structural problem in the back intensifies pain and fear and ensures that it will persist. This is the nocebo effect in action. Knowledge can reverse it.

Falling into the trap of the nocebo effect can hold you from seeking and accepting the knowledge necessary to return to health.

The Difference between the Placebo Effect and Knowledge

Healing from fibromyalgia is not a placebo effect; healing is based upon education about the *MindBodySpirit Connection* rather than upon blind faith. Enduring healing is based upon both faith and knowledge.

In the next chapter, you will learn how to partner with your doctor in order to facilitate healing.

Chapter 14

Consulting with Your Doctor

The witch doctor succeeds for the same reason all the rest of us succeed. Each patient carries his own doctor inside him. They come to us not knowing that truth. We are at our best when we give the doctor who resides within each patient a chance to go to work.
— Albert Schweitzer, M.D. (speaking to doctors)

A doctor who cannot take a good history and a patient who cannot give one are in danger of giving and receiving bad treatment.
— Paul Dudley White, M.D.

In his inspirational book on one's power to heal, *Head First: The Biology of Hope,* Norman Cousins said, "Belief becomes biology" (New York: E. P. Dutton, 1989). Another way of saying this is that what you believe in *mind* and *spirit* is manifested in the *body* through the *MindBodySpirit Connection.*

The Healing Placebo Effect or "Remembered Wellness"

Dr. Herbert Benson of Harvard University has emphasized that everyone has tremendous potential and power to heal through belief. Traditionally, this has been called the "placebo effect" as was discussed in the previous chapter, but Dr. Benson hopes to rename the placebo effect "remembered wellness," a way we can activate self-healing through faith. Dr. Benson also emphasizes how affirming beliefs, particularly belief in a higher power, contributes to physical health.

There are three components to "remembered wellness":

1. Belief and expectancy on the part of the patient
2. Belief and expectancy on the part of the caregiver (e.g., doctor)
3. Beliefs and expectancies generated by a relationship between the patient and the caregiver (e.g., doctor)

The placebo effect or "remembered wellness" is particularly important in the healing process. Eighty to ninety percent of symptoms and disorders that cause patients to consult with primary care physicians are best understood in the context of the *MindBodySpirit Connection* (Step 1).

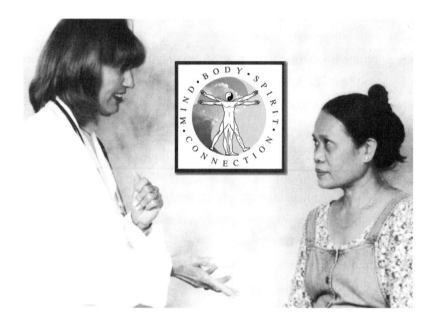

Belief Becomes Biology

This means that your own beliefs are very important in the healing process; but so are the beliefs of your doctor and the beliefs and expectancies of you both. So, find a caregiver who makes sense to you (someone you trust) and who is someone you believe can become your "partner" in your care.

The Doctor's Responsibility

Doctors try to determine why people have come to see them. Obviously, patients come to get a diagnosis and treatment. But sometimes the reason for the visit can be more complicated. The doctor needs to understand all of the reasons for your visit in order to help. We ask two questions of our patients in trying to diagnose and help them:

1. **What do you think is wrong with you?**   First of all, your opinion counts! Experience has taught us this important lesson: patients will often tell us the diagnosis if we will only allow them to do it! You should tell the doctor what you think is wrong with you, even if the question is not asked of you. We never cease to be amazed at how often patients really do seem to know what is wrong with them.

2. **What are your concerns about what might be wrong?**   This is a very different question, of course. It is important to determine the reason for the visit and what concerns or fears might be present in order to bring healing and relief. The most common concern or fear by far is that cancer might be present.

You learned about the nocebo effect in the last chapter. If you believe that you have a serious disease or cancer, then these negative beliefs interfere with healing.

Why People Visit a Doctor

Here are some of the reasons that people with fibromyalgia and other *MindBodySpirit Symptoms* decide to see the doctor:

- Severe symptoms, especially pain
- Recent stress
- Emotional problems, such as anxiety, depression, or a history of having been abused (mentally, physically, or sexually)
- An increased concern about having a serious disease (often because a family member or friend has received a serious diagnosis or has died)
- Impaired ability to perform at work or function in the family

- Belief that the problem has become disabling, or fear that it will become so
- Concern that others (usually family or coworkers) do not believe or understand how troubled or sick they are. In other words, patients feel the need to legitimize the illness.
- Unresolved losses. The death of a spouse, parent, or child, or operations with personal meaning (hysterectomy, ostomy, abortion, or stillbirth) can flare up or trigger symptoms of fibromyalgia, especially on the anniversaries of these events.

So, be sure to think carefully about why you have decided to see the doctor about your symptoms. If your doctor does not ask you, then volunteer your opinion about what you believe to be wrong and what your worries and concerns are. If you are worried about cancer—but the doctor does not suspect cancer based on your history, symptoms, and results of the examination—then you might not feel better if you fail to share your worry with him/her. If the doctor knows about your concern, then he/she can specifically address it.

In the next chapter, you will learn about the diseases and disorders that the doctor needs to consider before making the diagnosis of fibromyalgia.

Chapter 15
Differential Diagnosis of Fibromyalgia

The art consists in three things—the disease, the patient, and the physician. The physician is the servant of the art, and the patient must combat the disease along with the physician.
– Hippocrates (460–377? BC)

The symptoms of fibromyalgia, widespread musculoskeletal pain and fatigue, are very common and can be associated with several other syndromes, conditions, and diseases.

Why Differential Diagnosis Is Important

The differential diagnosis of fibromyalgia includes

- Identifying diseases that may mimic fibromyalgia so that they can be properly treated
- Recognizing that fibromyalgia often coexists (occurs with) these other diseases so that treatment can be directed to the fibromyalgia dimension of the problem
- Recognizing other *MindBodySpirit Symptoms* and *MindBodySpirit Syndromes* that often occur with fibromyalgia (discussed in Chapter 17)

Diseases That May Mimic Fibromyalgia

The symptoms of fibromyalgia, with generalized aching, pain, and fatigue can be confused with or mimic certain rheumatic and systemic illnesses that frequently affect younger women (Table 15.1). Treatment is then directed to the specific diagnosis.

Table 15.1

Differential Diagnoses and Systemic Disorders Associated with Fibromyalgia

Condition	Diagnostic Features
Osteoarthritis	Reduced joint range of motion, x-rays showing degenerative arthritis
Rheumatoid Arthritis	Inflamed, swollen joints (synovitis); blood tests showing elevated erythrocyte sedimentation rate (ESR), + rheumatoid factor
Sjogren's Syndrome	Swollen lymph nodes, biopsy of salivary glands
Systemic Lupus Erythematosis	Skin changes and blood vessel changes (vasculitis); blood tests with + ANA (antinuclear antibody)
Ankylosing Spondylitis	X-ray changes of sacroiliitis; blood tests with elevated erythrocyte sedimentation rate (ESR) and + HLA-B27 test
Polymyalgia Rheumatica (PMR)	Blood test: elevated erythrocyte sedimentation rate (ESR) and response to treatment with corticosteroids
Myositis and Myopathies	Blood test: increased muscle enzymes (CPK, aldolase)
Hypothyroidism	Blood test: abnormal thyroid function test—usually elevated TSH (thyroid stimulating hormone)
Cancer metastatic to bone	Blood test: elevated erythrocyte sedimentation rate (ESR); elevated alkaline phosphatase; x-ray and bone scan showing abnormal changes
Multiple Myeloma	Blood test: elevated erythrocyte sedimentation rate (ESR); abnormal serum protein electrophoresis (blood proteins); x-rays showing abnormal changes; abnormal bone marrow test

Fibromyalgia often coexists with the disorders listed in Table 15.1, like rheumatoid arthritis and osteoarthritis. Therefore, it can be quite difficult to determine whether the symptoms of pain and fatigue are a manifestation of fibromyalgia or a concurrent and coexisting disorder. Even if a disease is present, most of the symptoms may be attributed to fibromyalgia. So treatment is better directed to fibromyalgia than to the disease that coexists with fibromyalgia. The following are the important disorders and diseases that can either mimic fibromyalgia or coexist with it.

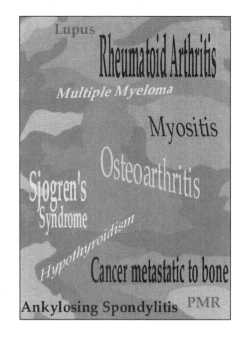

Osteoarthritis

Osteoarthritis is the most common rheumatic disorder affecting the joints. It is estimated that 12 percent of the population of the United States suffers from osteoarthritis, and it becomes more common with age. The cause of osteoarthritis remains unknown, but the cartilage within joints becomes damaged.

The main symptom of osteoarthritis is pain involving hips, knees, hands, fingers, neck, and back. Diagnosis is made by the physical examination and x-ray. Since it is very common for fibromyalgia and osteoarthritis to coexist, the diagnosis of osteoarthritis does not necessarily mean that the musculoskeletal pain is related. Furthermore, treatment is often better directed to the fibromyalgia that coexists.

Rheumatoid arthritis, Sjögren's syndrome, and systemic lupus erythematosus (SLE)

These systemic connective tissue diseases may coexist and also share symptoms of musculoskeletal pain and fatigue with fibromyalgia. Furthermore, Raynaud's phenomenon (fingers turning colors, particularly when exposed to cold weather) and sicca (dry eyes and dry mouth), which are classic features of these diseases, are present in 25 to 50 percent of patients with fibromyalgia.

A doctor can differentiate fibromyalgia from a connective tissue disease by careful history and physical examination and through blood tests when necessary. Muscles and joints are not inflamed in fibromyalgia.

It is usually important to use blood tests only when there is a reasonable concern that a disease process is present. Here is why. Approximately 10 percent of patients with fibromyalgia have a positive antinuclear antibody (ANA) test. But 5 to 10 percent of healthy women also have a positive ANA titer. So a positive ANA does not necessarily translate into a diagnosis of SLE without actual symptoms and findings on physical examination typical of the disease. If uncertainty remains relative to the differential diagnosis of fibromyalgia and SLE, more specific (and expensive) blood tests, such as an anti-DNA antibody test, can be obtained.

Ankylosing spondylitis

Inflammatory back conditions like ankylosing spondylitis can be associated with musculoskeletal pain and stiffness similar to that of fibromyalgia. But spinal motion is restricted in these disorders, while it is generally normal in fibromyalgia. Furthermore, typical x-ray changes of ankylosing spondylitis and the other seronegative spondyloarthropathies are absent in fibromyalgia.

Polymyalgia rheumatica (PMR)

Polymyalgia rheumatica may mimic fibromyalgia, although this disorder can be differentiated by the history and laboratory tests in the following four areas:

- Tender points have not been consistently reported in patients with PMR.
- Stiffness is more prominent than pain in patients with PMR.
- Most with PMR have an elevated ESR (erythrocyte sedimentation rate) blood test, while the ESR is normal in patients with fibromyalgia.
- Patients with PMR respond extremely well to modest doses of corticosteroids like prednisone, while those with fibromyalgia do not.

Corticosteroid withdrawal

Steroid withdrawal in PMR or any rheumatic condition or disease may cause symptoms that are similar to those of fibromyalgia for several weeks to months.

Inflammatory myositis and metabolic myopathies

Fibromyalgia is distinguished from inflammatory myositis (muscle inflammation) and the metabolic myopathies (muscle diseases) by the following features:

- Myositis and the myopathies cause muscle weakness and muscle fatigue but are not usually associated with diffuse pain.
- Muscle weakness is not usually present in patients with fibromyalgia other than that associated with pain and deconditioning.
- Patients with fibromyalgia have normal muscle enzyme tests (like CPK or aldolase) and normal or nondiagnostic findings on muscle biopsy, in contrast to those with myositis or myopathy. Muscle biopsy is not necessary unless there is evidence of muscle inflammation or abnormality.

Hypothyroidism

Patients who have hypothyroidism, or an underactive thyroid state, often have generalized aches, fatigue, and sleep disturbance—all of the symptoms of fibromyalgia. So thyroid blood tests are part of the routine initial evaluation of a patient with suspected fibromyalgia.

Hypothyroidism may be difficult to distinguish from fibromyalgia because patients with hypothyroidism often complain of generalized aches, fatigue, and interrupted sleep. Thus, thyroid function studies (usually a serum TSH level) are usually obtained during the initial evaluation of a patient with suspected fibromyalgia. Both fibromyalgia and hypothyroidism are common, so they often occur together. If so, then correction of the thyroid abnormality will not relieve the symptoms of fibromyalgia.

Other endocrine disorders

Other endocrine disorders, hyperparathyroidism and Cushing's syndrome, may present with fibromyalgia-like symptoms. Hyperparathyroidism is recognized by the presence of hypercalcemia (elevated calcium in the blood), while Cushing's syndrome is accompanied by typical facial and skin features and is associated with muscle weakness rather than pain.

Peripheral neuropathies, entrapment syndromes (pinched nerve), and neurologic disorders

Peripheral neuropathies, entrapment syndromes (such as carpal tunnel syndrome), and neurologic disorders (such as multiple sclerosis and myasthenia gravis) can mimic fibromyalgia. Fibromyalgia patients are commonly misdiagnosed with one of these disorders because they may complain of numbness and tingling, often involving the neck and radiating down the arm, suggesting cervical radiculopathy (pinched nerve). These symptoms of numbness and tingling, called paresthesias, as well as subjective cognitive dysfunction—the sense that memory and thinking are impaired—can result in expensive and uncomfortable neurologic testing. A careful neurologic examination should permit the differentiation of fibromyalgia from neurologic disease. So, unless there is evidence of nerve compression or cervical or lumbar spinal stenosis (narrowing), extensive testing including x-rays, electromyography (EMG), nerve conduction velocities, CT scans, nuclear scans, or MRI is not usually necessary.

Infections

Fibromyalgia has been noted to follow well-documented infections, including human immunodeficiency virus (HIV) infection and Lyme disease. About ⅓ of patients with documented Lyme disease treated with appropriate antibiotics develop persistent pain and fatigue typical of fibromyalgia and chronic fatigue syndrome. But, there is no scientific evidence of persistent infection in most of these patients. Also, antibiotics are not effective in this "post-Lyme" fibromyalgia/CFS condition.

Cancer and multiple myeloma

Occasionally, patients with bone cancer will consult with a doctor for what appears to be a fibromyalgia-like illness. However, this is rare, and there are other clues to the presence of a serious disease, such as loss of appetite, involuntary weight loss, fever, and night sweats.

Fibromyalgia Along with Other Disorders and Illnesses

Fibromyalgia commonly coexists along with other disorders and diseases. For example, it is common to have both osteoarthritis and fibromyalgia. Understanding this is important for two reasons. First, the presence of a structural finding does not necessarily mean that it is causing any symptoms or trouble. In the osteoarthritis/fibromyalgia example, the presence of osteoarthritis on x-ray is not necessarily an explanation for pain. It is common to find osteoarthritis on x-ray that is not causing any symptoms or pain. You have already learned that falsely attributing the pain of fibromyalgia to osteoarthritis can interfere with the healing process.

Second, treatment may be directed to the disorder or disease that coexists with fibromyalgia rather than to the culprit: fibromyalgia. So, strong treatment and medication may be used that may cause side effects and be unnecessary. Furthermore, the opportunity to treat fibromyalgia may be missed, or at the very least, delayed.

Different *MindBodySpirit Symptoms* and *MindBodySpirit Syndromes* commonly occur together. This is discussed further in Chapter 17.

You will learn how fibromyalgia is diagnosed in the next chapter.

Chapter 16

Diagnosis of Fibromyalgia: Widespread Muscular Pain and Trigger (Tender) Points

It is of the highest importance in the art of detection to recognize out of a number of facts, which are incidental and which are vital.
– Sherlock Holmes, as quoted by
Sir Arthur Conan Doyle (1859–1930)

It is important to obtain a correct diagnosis in order to begin healing.

Definition of Fibromyalgia

In Chapter 9, you learned that the definition of fibromyalgia is widespread muscular aching and stiffness associated with tenderness on palpation at specified sites called tender points. Otherwise, the physical examination and any other tests that may be done (like blood tests and x-rays) are completely normal.

Pain Location

Pain can be located at the base of the skull, in the neck, shoulders, chest, back, arms, legs, buttocks, or hips. Refer to Table 9.1 in Chapter 9.

Diagnosis of Fibromyalgia

The diagnosis of fibromyalgia is based upon the exclusion of disorders and diseases that may mimic the condition (Chapter 15) and the presence of clinical criteria (Table 16.1 and Figure 16.1).

Table 16.1

Diagnostic Criteria for Fibromyalgia*

- Widespread pain with pain on the right and left side of the body and both above and below the waist
- Pain on palpation with the thumb or forefinger at 11 of 18 known trigger (tender) points

*According to the American College of Rheumatology.

Trigger (Tender) Points

In 1990, the American College of Rheumatology (ACR) published criteria for the diagnosis of fibromyalgia. The results of a multicenter clinical study indicated that the presence of 11 or more out of 18 trigger or tender points associated with a history of widespread musculoskeletal pain provided the best diagnostic sensitivity for fibromyalgia. These trigger or tender points are shown in Figure 16.1. These points are palpated with moderate pressure using the pulp of the thumb or forefinger.

Although the ACR criteria call for the examination of 18 points, many fibromyalgia patients have multiple tender points in other locations and many with typical fibromyalgia symptoms have fewer than 11 tender points. This means that fibromyalgia can be diagnosed if unexplained widespread muscular pain is present, regardless of whether 11 trigger points are actually identified.

Dermatographia

The skin is often hypersensitive to scratching with the finger so that red marks form. This "skin writing" is called dermatographia and can

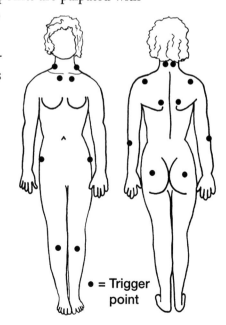

• = Trigger point

Figure 16.1

look like someone could play tic tac toe on your back. This skin hyper-sensitivity is thought to be related to an overactive sympathetic nervous system. The dermatographia is most prominent in the skin that overlies the painful muscles.

Blood Tests

Some baseline blood tests are usually obtained, including

- Complete blood count
- Erythrocyte sedimentation rate
- Standard blood chemistries (also known as a multichemistry, SMA-12, or SMAC)
- Muscle enzymes
- Thyroid function blood tests

These tests are all usually normal in patients with fibromyalgia, so any abnormalities could suggest the presence of one of the systemic diseases discussed in the previous chapter (Chapter 15).

Most patients who have fibromyalgia have other *MindBodySpirit Symptoms* and *MindBodySpirit Syndromes* which overlap, and you will learn about this in the next chapter.

Chapter 17

MindBodySpirit Symptoms and Syndromes Associated with Fibromyalgia

> The human body is far more robust than people have been led to believe. Public education in health matters has tended to make people overestimate their weaknesses and underestimate their strengths. The result is that we are in danger of becoming a nation of weaklings and hypochondriacs.
>
> *– Head First: The Biology of Hope*
> Norman Cousins

Most people who consult doctors for fibromyalgia have multiple *MindBodySpirit Symptoms* that cannot be explained by tests and science. These people become patients who are diagnosed with *MindBodySpirit Syndromes.*

MindBodySpirit Symptoms

You now know that *MindBodySpirit Symptoms* affect everyone and that they are the most common symptoms that cause people to consult with doctors. They are listed in Table 2 in the introduction, *Your Prescription for Change!,* and include fatigue, headache, and unexplained pain anywhere in the *body.*

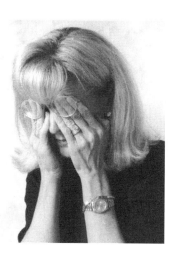

MindBodySpirit Syndromes

In Step 1, you learned that when people with these *MindBodySpirit Symptoms* consult with doctors, they become patients and are diagnosed with *MindBodySpirit Syndromes,* which are collections of symptoms that cannot be explained by tests. The syndrome diagnosis depends upon the predominant symptoms and the type of specialist seen (Table 17.1). Many have seen more than one specialist and received more than one diagnosis of an illness and syndrome.

Table 17.1	
Specialist Diagnosis of MindBodySpirit Symptoms	
Specialist	**Diagnosis**
Rheumatologist or orthopedic surgeon	Fibromyalgia (FMS)
Infectious disease specialist	Chronic fatigue syndrome (CFS)
Sleep specialist	Sleep disorder
Psychiatrist	Depression; anxiety; somatoform disorder
Neurologist	Tension headache or migraine syndrome
Dentist	Temporomandibular joint (TMJ) syndrome
Cardiologist	Chest pain, normal coronary arteries
Gastroenterologist	Irritable bowel syndrome (IBS); functional dyspepsia; chronic functional abdominal pain (CFAP)
Urologist	Interstitial cystitis or female urethral syndrome (irritable bladder syndrome)
Gynecologist	Primary dysmenorrhea; premenstrual tension syndrome (PMS); chronic pelvic pain syndrome
Allergist	Multiple chemical sensitivity syndrome

Dr. Muhammad Yunus, M.D., rheumatologist and fibromyalgia re-searcher from the University of Illinois College of Medicine, states that many if not most people who consult with a doctor about functional *body* symptoms *(MindBodySpirit Symptoms)* have more than one syn-drome *(MindBodySpirit Syndrome)*. Other researchers who seem to have a similar view include Dedra Buchwald, M.D., of the University of Wash-ington; Robert Bennett, M.D., of Oregon Health Sciences University in Portland; Anthony Komaroff, M.D., of Brigham and Women's Hospital in Boston; Don Goldenberg, M.D., of Newton-Wellesley Hospital in Boston; Herbert Benson, M.D., of Harvard; John Sarno, M.D., of New York University School of Medicine; and Kurt Kroenke, M.D., of the University of Indiana.

Dysregulation spectrum syndrome

Dr. Yunus views fibromyalgia and chronic fatigue syndrome as part of a larger spectrum of conditions, which he calls dysregulation spectrum syn-drome (DSS). The dysregulation spectrum syndrome is depicted in Figure 17.1. The term "dysregulation" is used to mean "biophysiological abnor-malities," at least in part related to the way the brain and body communi-cate through the nervous system, glandular system (endocrine system), and by way of chemicals that relay information throughout the body (neuro-transmitters). The *mind* (brain) seems to have a problem processing sensa-tions from the *body* with an increase in sensitivity.

Think of dysregulation spectrum syndrome as another term for *Mind-BodySpirit Syndromes*.

The MindBodySpirit Connection

You may want to refer back to Chapter 8 for our reasons for proposing the new language of the *MindBodySpirit Connection*. This modern and inclusive terminology and language will help people, patients, and doc-tors communicate with one another about these very real *MindBodySpirit Symptoms* and *MindBodySpirit Syndromes* for a common purpose: healing.

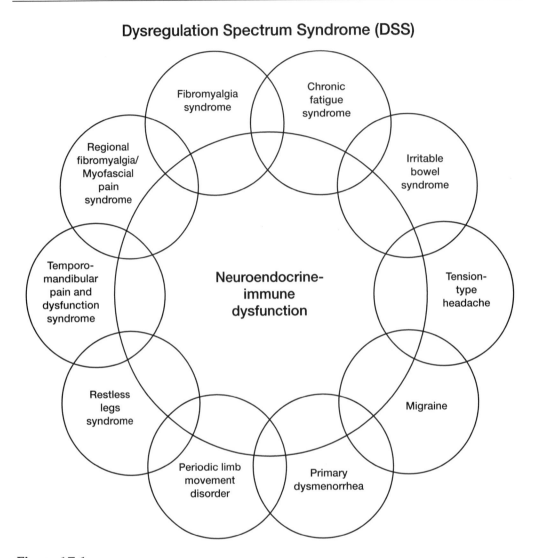

Figure 17.1
Reproduced with permission from Yunus MB, Baillieres Rheumatology 1994; 8:811–37.

Specific MindBodySpirit Symptoms and MindBodySpirit Syndromes

Three *MindBodySpirit Symptoms* and *MindBodySpirit Syndromes* that may be of interest to people with fibromyalgia are

- **Myofascial pain and temporomandibular joint dysfunction**
  These are localized forms of fibromyalgia, which are discussed in Chapter 10.

- **Sleep disturbance**   Problems with sleeping are almost always present in fibromyalgia. Sleep is discussed in Chapter 25.

- **Fatigue and chronic fatigue syndrome (CFS)**   Most who have fibromyalgia also suffer with the symptom of fatigue. Furthermore, chronic fatigue syndrome (CFS), which is a *MindBodySpirit Syndrome,* shares many similar features with fibromyalgia.

People have suffered with unexplained fatigue for centuries. Over the years, many terms and syndromes have been used to describe the illness (Table 17.2).

Table 17.2

Synonyms for the Chronic Fatigue Syndrome

Febricula	Hypoglycemia
Nervous exhaustion	"Total allergy" syndrome
Neurasthenia	Chronic candidiasis
DaCosta's syndrome	Chronic Epstein Barr virus infection
Effort syndrome	
Autonomic imbalance syndrome	Chronic fatigue syndrome
Chronic brucellosis	Chronic fatigue and immune dysfunction syndrome

---

From Bennett, R.M.: The fibromyalgia syndrome: myofascial pain and the chronic fatigue syndrome, in Kelley, W. (ed.), *Textbook of Rheumatology, 4th edition,* Philadelphia, W.B. Saunders Co., 1993.

Most people who consult doctors with the symptom of fatigue do not have chronic fatigue syndrome (CFS). However, it is important to stress that fibromyalgia and CFS share similar clinical features. The diagnosis of CFS is described in Table 17.3.

Table 17.3

Chronic Fatigue Syndrome
Case Definition Symptom Criteria

To fulfill the case definition, severe fatigue of new onset and four or more of the following symptoms must be present concurrently for at least 6 months:

- Impaired memory or concentration
- Sore throat
- Tender cervical or axillary lymph nodes
- Muscle pain
- Multijoint pain
- New headaches
- Unrefreshing sleep
- Postexertion malaise

From Fukuda K, Straus SE, Hickie I, et.al., for the International Chronic Fatigue Syndrome Study Group. *The chronic fatigue syndrome: a comprehensive approach to its definition and study.* Annals of Internal Medicine. 1994;121:953–959.

Many patients with CFS have chronic musculoskeletal pain and a sleep disturbance. Most of these people can be diagnosed with fibromyalgia according to current diagnostic criteria (see Chapter 16 and Table 16.1). These *MindBodySpirit Symptoms* and *MindBodySpirit Syndromes* all overlap through the *MindBodySpirit Connection.*

In the next chapter, we will dispel some common myths and misunderstandings about fibromyalgia.

Chapter 18
Dispelling Myths about Fibromyalgia

I therefore claim to show, not how men think in myths, but how
myths operate in men's minds without their being aware of the fact.
– *The Raw and the Cooked, "Overture," sct. 1* (1964)
Claude Levi-Strauss (French anthropologist)

There are several common myths and misunderstandings about
fibromyalgia.

Myth: The pain is all in my head or is caused by an emotional disturbance.
There is nothing imaginary about the pain and symptoms of fibromyalgia. But it is important to understand that the problem is related to the
linkage and interaction of your *mind, body,* and *spirit.* You have the power
to heal by understanding the *MindBodySpirit Connection.*

Myth: Fibromyalgia can lead to cancer.
There is no increase in risk of developing cancer from fibromyalgia.

Myth: It's all caused by stress and anxiety.
Stress affects all human illnesses and conditions and does play an important role in fibromyalgia.

Myth: I will need a lot of tests to find out what is wrong.
The diagnosis of fibromyalgia can be made on physical examination and
after finding that certain simple blood tests are normal.

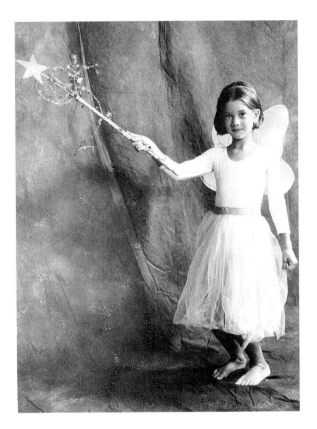

Myth: Fibromyalgia is a form of arthritis.

Fibromyalgia is not related to arthritis. But many people with arthritis also have fibromyalgia. So treating the fibromyalgia can bring improvement even when arthritis is present.

Myth: Fibromyalgia can lead to deterioration or deformity of my body.

Fibromyalgia will not affect how long you live or the appearance of your body. Fibromyalgia does not increase the risk of developing any serious disease or disorder.

Myth: My muscles are inflammed and abnormal.

The muscles are normal in fibromyalgia. There is no evidence of inflammation on physical examination and blood testing.

Myth: Fibromyalgia is caused by a chronic infection or trauma.

Even if an infection, accident, or injury triggers or aggravates symptoms, there is no scientific evidence of ongoing undiagnosed infection or trauma.

Myth: My doctor has told me that fibromyalgia does not exist.

Fibromyalgia is a real symptom complex and illness and is not imagined. The symptoms are *MindBodySpirit Symptoms*. Fibromyalgia is a *MindBodySpirit Syndrome*. Fibromyalgia can be understood through the *MindBodySpirit Connection*.

Myth: I cannot live a normal and healthy life with fibromyalgia.

You have more power and control over your body than you may realize. Simply acknowledging that the cause(s) can only be understood through the *MindBodySpirit Connection* can be therapeutic. You can heal.

Take the next step to make the *"Connection."*

REVIEW OF STEP 3

1. The difference between healing and treatment is that treatment originates from without, while healing comes from within.

2. Belief in a treatment may bring relief of symptoms, even if the treatment has not been scientifically proven to be of value. This is called, the "placebo effect." Conversely, negative belief, or the "nocebo effect," can have a harmful effect.

3. Your own beliefs are very important in the healing process; however, so are the beliefs of your doctor and the beliefs and expectancies of you both.

4. Differential diagnosis of fibromyalgia is important for the following reasons:
   • Identifying diseases that may mimic fibromyalgia so that they can be properly treated
   • Confirming that fibromyalgia often coexists, or occurs with, these other diseases so that treatment can be directed to the fibromyalgia dimension of the problem
   • Recognizing other *MindBodySpirit Symptoms* and *MindBodySpirit Syndromes* that often occur with fibromyalgia

5. The diagnosis of fibromyalgia is based upon the exclusion of disorders and diseases that may mimic the condition and the presence of clinical criteria (American College of Rheumatology Diagnostic Criteria for Fibromyalgia):
   • Widespread pain with pain on the right and left side of the body and both above and below the waist
   • Pain on palpation with the thumb or forefinger at 11 of 18 known trigger (tender) points

6. Most people who consult doctors for fibromyalgia have multiple *MindBodySpirit Symptoms* that cannot be explained by tests and science. These people become patients and are diagnosed with a *MindBodySpirit Syndrome.* Examples include chronic fatigue syn-

drome, irritable bowel syndrome, chronic headache syndromes, and irritable bladder syndrome.

7. There are several common myths and misunderstandings about fibromyalgia.

STEP 4

MAKING "THE CONNECTION"

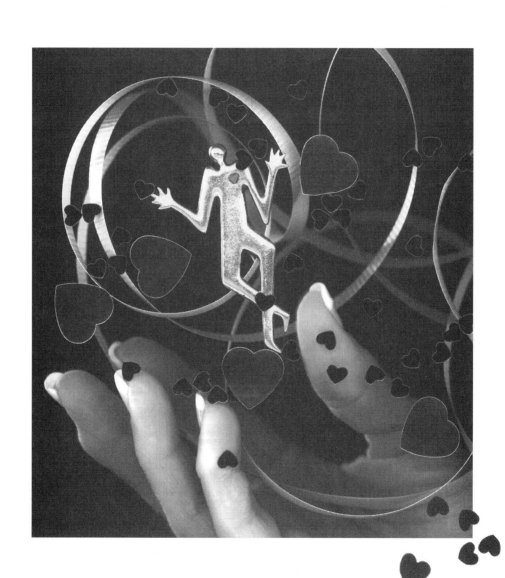

Chapter 19

Self-Tests for Personal and Emotional Problems

No wind serves him who addresses his voyage to no certain point.
— Seneca

Anxiety cannot be avoided, but it can be reduced.
— Rollo May

Distress and pain are friends to growth.
— Augustus Napier

> You can make the *"Connection"* and step toward healing by accepting that perceived stress, emotional distress, memory, and thought affect and influence whether and to what extent and degree you experience symptoms, whether you feel ill or unwell with them, whether you miss work or social opportunities, and whether you report them to doctors.

Drugs

First, consider the possibility that a drug, medication, or substance (like recreational drugs, nicotine, or caffeine) could be contributing to or aggravating unpleasant symptoms like pain, fatigue, sleeplessness, anxiety, and depression (Chapter 31). For example, caffeine is a stimulant that can contribute to anxiety and aggravate symptoms.

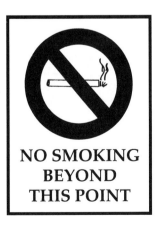

**NO SMOKING
BEYOND
THIS POINT**

Self-Assessment Screening

Here are five self-assessment "screens" that we have compiled so you can determine if a personal problem, harmful stress, emotional distress, or painful memories could be important factors in your fibromyalgia. You should not use these screens to diagnose yourself. Your doctor needs to confirm any diagnosis with additional questioning and evaluation. Still, this information may alert you to the possible presence of a problem and prompt you to see a doctor. It should help you to be a real partner in diagnosis and treatment and to assume responsibility for your recovery.

Alcohol abuse and alcoholism

Alcohol is the most commonly abused drug in the world. In the United States, alcohol is used by at least one-half of the adult population. Alcoholism affects up to 10 percent of the population, up to 20 percent of people who go to see doctors, and 10 to 40 percent of hospitalized patients. Alcohol is responsible for 100,000 deaths every year, and estimated costs to people and society are approximately $130 billion.

Alcoholism can contribute to the symptoms of fibromyalgia (Chapter 31). Furthermore, alcoholism is associated with anxiety, depression, and other emotional problems. Doctors detect drinking problems in as few as 35% of patients who have them because most deny having a problem with alcohol.

What is moderation in alcohol?

The new and updated *"Dietary Guidelines for Americans"* recommended by the federal government has changed relative to alcohol (*Nutrition and Your Health: Dietary Guidelines for Americans.* Fourth Edition, 1995; U.S. Department of Agriculture and U.S. Department of Health and Human Services). Previous guidelines have denied that drinking held any benefits, but the new guidelines acknowledge that "alcoholic beverages have been used to enhance the enjoyment of meals by many societies," and cite recent scientific studies that suggest that moderate drinkers seem to have reduced rates of heart disease. The guidelines conclude, "If you drink, do so in moderation."

Definition of moderation

Moderation means no more than one drink per day for women and no more than two drinks per day for men.

Count as a drink:
- 12 ounces of regular beer (150 calories)
- 5 ounces of wine (100 calories)
- 1.5 ounces of 80-proof distilled spirits (100 calories)

A screen for alcohol abuse

Two questions

If you answer "yes" to either of these two questions, then you could have a problem with alcohol:

1. Have you ever had a drinking problem before?
2. Do you have more than two drinks on most days if you are man or more than one drink on most days if you are a woman?

The CAGE questionnaire

Here is a simple screen for alcoholism.

1. Have you ever felt the need to	Cut down on your drinking?
2. Have you ever felt	Annoyed by criticism of your drinking?
3. Have you ever had	Guilty feelings about drinking?
4. Have you ever taken a morning	Eye-opener?

(From Ewing JA. *Detecting alcoholism: the CAGE questionnaire;* Journal of the American Medical Association. 1984;252:1905–7.)

The more questions answered "yes," the more likely you have a problem with alcohol.

A screen for depression

You have learned how common it is for people to consult with doctors because of symptoms related to perceived stress and emotional distress.

Most people with depression do not come to the doctor announcing, "Doctor, I am sad and depressed." Instead, they report real *body* symptoms, such as abdominal pain, headaches, fatigue, and sleeplessness.

Here is a brief screen that may allow you to recognize depression in yourself. If you answer yes to five or more of these questions (including questions #1 and #2) and the symptoms have been present nearly every day for two weeks or more, then you may be depressed.

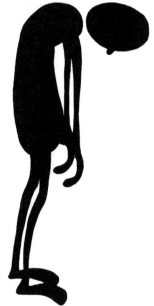

1. Do you feel a deep sense of sadness, hopelessness, or feeling "down" most of the day?
2. Have you noticed a loss of interest or pleasure in doing most things and in most activities?
3. Have you had a significant change in appetite or weight (up or down) when not dieting?
4. Have you had a significant change in sleeping patterns (trouble falling or remaining asleep, or too much sleeping)?
5. Do you feel especially restless and fidgety, or do you feel especially tired and sluggish?
6. Do you feel unusually fatigued with low energy?
7. Do you feel badly about yourself, that you are a failure, have let other people down, are worthless, or feel guilty about things?
8. Have you had trouble thinking and concentrating, or difficulty making decisions?
9. Do you have recurrent thoughts of hurting yourself, death, or committing suicide?

(Adapted from the *Diagnostic and Statistical Manual of Mental Disorders, Fourth Edition.* Copyright 1994 American Psychiatric Association.)

A screen for anxiety and panic

It is estimated that over ten million Americans have persistent anxiety that can cause or contribute to significant mental and physical symptoms.

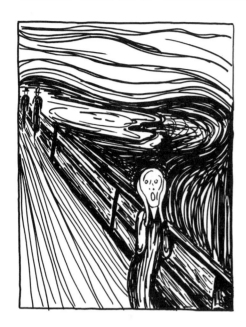

Generalized anxiety disorder (GAD)

Here is a brief screen for a generalized anxiety disorder, which may allow you to check for anxiety in yourself.

Have you been troubled on most days for more than six months with excessive and unrealistic worry that you feel you cannot control? If you have, do you also suffer from three or more of the following symptoms?

1. Irritability
2. Muscle tension
3. Restlessness, feeling keyed up or on edge
4. Fatigue
5. Difficulty with concentration or with your mind going blank
6. Sleep problems (difficulty falling or remaining asleep or restless sleep that does not restore energy)

(Adapted from the *Diagnostic and Statistical Manual of Mental Disorders, Fourth Edition.* Copyright 1994 American Psychiatric Association.)

Panic attack and panic disorder

A panic attack is a type of anxiety characterized by an unprovoked episode or explosion of bodily sensations, symptoms, and fear which usually lasts just a few minutes to several hours. The American Psychiatric Association defines a panic attack as an unprovoked surge of fear accompanied by at least four of the following physical and emotional symptoms (although a limited symptom panic attack can occur with fewer than four symptoms):

- Shortness of breath or smothering sensations
- Dizziness or faintness
- Accelerated heart rate
- Trembling or shaking
- Sweating
- Choking

- Nausea or abdominal distress
- Feelings of detachment or unreality
- Chest discomfort or pain
- Numbness or tingling sensations
- Hot flashes or chills
- A fear of dying, going crazy, or losing control

Sudden and intense anxiety triggered by situations where a person fears being the focus of others' attention is not considered a true panic attack.

The difference between a panic attack and a panic disorder

The difference between a panic attack and panic disorder is the frequency of attacks or their emotional impact. A panic disorder is diagnosed if four or more panic attacks occur within any four-week period, or if fewer than four attacks are followed by a month of persistent fear of having another attack.

A screen for a somatoform disorder

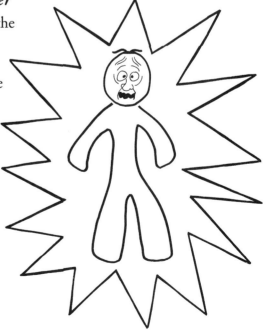

Somatization is the *body* expression of the effects of stress, emotional distress, and psychological problems (Step 1). When these symptoms repeatedly cause people to see doctors and interfere with living, the condition is called a *somatoform disorder.* Medical tests are normal and do not explain the many *body* symptoms of a somatoform disorder. The symptoms have usually been present or recurring for a long time, often for years. You can think of a somatoform disorder as a psychiatric diagnosis of *MindBodySpirit Symptoms* and *MindBodySpirit Syndromes.*

Since many of the symptoms of a somatoform disorder are also symptoms of other illnesses, many tests and medical evaluations may have already been done to assure that no other disorder or disease is present.

The symptoms of somatization and a somatoform disorder include:

- Digestive symptoms like nausea, gas, indigestion, abdominal pain, bloating, constipation, loose stools or diarrhea
- Fatigue
- Difficulty sleeping
- Headaches
- Dizziness
- Feeling faint or fainting
- Chest pain
- Back pain
- Menstrual pain
- Bladder symptoms
- Pain with sexual intercourse
- Pain in the arms, legs, or joints (like shoulders, hips, knees)
- Heart pounding or racing
- Shortness of breath

A somatoform disorder could be present if (1) there are three or more of these physical symptoms that have interfered considerably with life and activities in the last month, and (2) medical tests have been unable to explain the symptoms.

A screen for an eating disorder

Particularly in adolescent girls, the perceived need to gain control over one's life can express itself as an eating disorder, either anorexia nervosa (not eating enough) or bulimia nervosa (self-induced vomiting). Young women often view themselves as heavy even when they are not overweight. There are unrealistic body appearance and weight standards in American society set by advertising and fashion models. People are led to believe that they should be thin—perhaps very thin. If one's self-esteem is low and opportunities for assertiveness have been limited, the discovery that attention can be gained by altering the body can be powerful and eye opening. In order to maintain attention, a person with an eating disorder may continue to lose weight through a combination of continuous dieting, exercise, and self-induced vomiting, or use of laxatives and diuretics.

If the answer to any of these four questions is "yes," then you could have an eating disorder:

1. Do you have a problem with eating and/or weight control?
2. Do you ever throw up after eating?
3. Do you ever overeat when anxious and then throw up afterward?
4. Do you make yourself vomit or do you take laxatives to keep from gaining weight or to lose weight?

Remember, you should confirm with a doctor any problem or diagnosis that you might suspect as a result of the screens in this chapter.

In the next chapter, you will learn how to use a symptom diary to help you find the way to healing.

Chapter 20

Keeping a Journal

Memory…is the diary that we all carry about with us.
— *The Importance of Being Earnest*
Oscar Wilde

It does not matter how slowly you go, so long as you do not stop.
— Confucius

It is not simply mind over matter, but it is clear that mind matters.
— *Journal of the American Medical Association;* April 14, 1999
David Spiegel, M.D.

Confessional writing has been advocated since the Renaissance, but new research has demonstrated that writing about emotionally traumatic experiences has a surprisingly beneficial effect on health.

Biopsychosocialspiritual Model, Emotion, Thoughts, and Stress

In the first step of this book, you learned about the importance of psychological, social, and spiritual factors in understanding illness. Adverse emotional events range from major stressors to lesser ones that accumulate over time. These stressors may be perceived by conscious *mind* or not perceived and affect unconscious *mind.* You have also seen how the effects of accumulated stress can lead to an abnormal central stress response in the *mind* (brain). This translates into an enhanced sensitivity of the *body* and unpleasant symptoms, such as those experienced with fibromyalgia.

By contrast, social connection can have a positive and buffering effect upon stress. You have learned about the benefits of social support, love and connection with others, and spirituality.

Illness without Disease and Writing

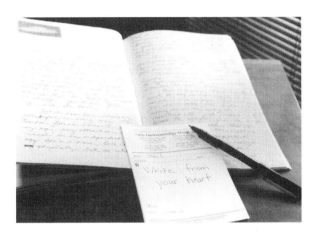

Evidence is accumulating that resilience to stress—even distress related to disease—is associated with how people manage their emotions. Finding meaning while enduring a distressing situation has been linked with a positive psychological state. Realistic optimism can be helpful, but so is dealing directly with a negative effect. In other words, the suppression of negative emotion can reduce a person's ability to experience any emotion, whether it be positive or negative. Research has demonstrated that expressive writing about emotionally traumatic experiences can have a surprisingly beneficial effect upon health for those who have illness without disease in terms of symptom reduction, sense of well being, and diminished need to see a doctor.

Disease and Writing

A recent scientific study published in the *Journal of the American Medical Association* is the first to show that writing about stressful life experiences improves symptoms of disease (1999;281:1304–1309). Patients with either asthma or rheumatoid arthritis were asked to write for twenty minutes on three consecutive days about the most stressful experience that they had ever undergone. Half had reduced symptoms and objective evidence of reduction in disease severity when evaluated 4 months later. It is not clear if beneficial effects will endure beyond 4 months and if these results may be extended to other diseases. Still, these results will prompt more studies on the effects of structured writing and disease.

Write Off Pain

The release of negative emotion through the ventilation of writing to an unknown reader can help with the recognition and management of stress and distress and bring symptom relief. We offer you three suggestions for expressive writing.

1. Write about the most stressful experience that you have ever undergone. As you have just learned, this could help you to find symptom relief and feel better.
2. Ask yourself, "Was there something that happened in my life before the fibromyalgia began?" Or ask, "What was going on when my symptoms got worse?" Think carefully and be honest with yourself. Raising these questions and writing about them can help you to identify any relationship of your fibromyalgia to a life experience that you may not have realized relates to your illness.
3. Keep a daily journal for several weeks. This is an excellent way for you to learn and heal through the *MindBodySpirit Connection.* Keeping a journal can help you to emphasize your responsibility and power to heal and identify the relationship of your symptoms to thoughts, stress, emotion, memory, and life events. It may also assist both you and your doctor in helping you to find new ways to healing.

The journal in this chapter should be photocopied. Use one journal sheet every day for at least 4 weeks. Here are instructions on how to construct your journal.

Symptoms

Rate the severity of your pain and fatigue from 0 to 10, with 0 being no symptoms and 10 being the worst possible symptoms. For example, pain rated as "2" would be very mild, while pain rated "9" would be very severe. If you have other symptoms, list them and rate their severity. Rate your sleep as either good, fair, poor, or none.

Date: _____

Fibromyalgia Journal

		MORNING	AFTERNOON	EVENING	NIGHT
Symptoms Record severity on a scale of 1–10: 0 = None 10 = Unbearable	Pain				
	Fatigue				
	Other				Sleep: Good/Fair/Poor/None
Mind and Life My thoughts, emotions, stresses, memories, and what is happening in my life					
Analysis My impression of any relationship of my symptoms to my *mind* and life					
Reprogramming* Write one statement each day.					

*See list of reprogramming statements on p. 118.

Mind and life

Describe your thoughts, emotions, stresses, memories, and what is happening in your life. This may permit you to recognize a correlation with your symptoms and fibromyalgia illness.

Analysis

Review your journal at least daily and more frequently if possible. In the space provided, evaluate your findings, observations, and draw conclusions. It is important to record not only your observations, but also your impressions about any relationship of your symptoms to your *mind* and life. Look for patterns and try to draw conclusions.

Reprogramming statements

Each of the following statements will help you to make the *"Connection"* and reprogram negative thoughts into positive ones. Put them in a place where you will see them often, and read them daily. Write a different one down each day until all seven are recorded, and memorize them if you wish. Do this each week that you keep the journal. Here are the reprogramming statements.

1. My *mind, body,* and *spirit* are one. Their *Connection* cannot be broken.
2. Everyone experiences *MindBodySpirit Symptoms,* and millions of people are diagnosed with *MindBodySpirit Syndromes.*
3. My fibromyalgia is a *MindBodySpirit Syndrome;* although it is an illness rather than a disease, it is not a mental illness.
4. My fibromyalgia is related in some way—at least in part—to perceived stress, emotional distress, memory, and thoughts, and I have nothing to be ashamed of here.
5. I now realize that understanding and accepting the *MindBodySpirit Connection* will help me to cope with my fibromyalgia, to recover, and to heal.
6. I understand the difference between treatment and healing; I acknowledge my power to heal and accept responsibility for my health.
7. I will "use" my illness, fibromyalgia, to change myself and become healthier than ever before.

Resources

If you are interested in more information about keeping a journal and expressive writing, here are several resources.

Books

- Adams, Kathleen. *Journal to the Self.* Warner Books, 1990.
- DeSalvo, Louise. *Writing as a Way of Healing: How Telling Our Stories Transforms Our Lives.* Harper San Francisco, 1999.
- Pennebaker, James W. *Opening Up: The Healing Power of Expressing Emotions.* Guilford Press, 1997.

Internet

- Smyth JM, Stone AA, Hurewitz A, Kaell A. Effects of writing about stressful experiences on symptom reduction in patients with asthma or rheumatoid arthritis. *Journal of the American Medical Association.* 1999;281:1304–1309. The full text of this article may be found at the Web site of the American Medical Association www.ama-assn.org. The specific link is www.ama-assn.org/special/asthma/library/readroom/pc90005.htm.
- Spiegel D. Healing words: emotional expression and disease outcome. *Journal of the American Medical Association.* 1999;281:1328–1329. This is a related editorial to the previous article by Smyth. The full text of the article is also available at www.ama-assn.org. The specific link is www.ama-assn.org/special/asthma/library/readroom/ed90017x.htm.
- Center for Journal Therapy (Kathleen Adams) www.journaltherapy.com (888) 421-2298

In the next chapter, you will learn how to manage stress.

Chapter 21

Stress Management and Relaxation Techniques

We boil at different degrees.
– *Society and Solitude* (1870)
Ralph Waldo Emerson

Breath is the link between the body and mind and between
the conscious and unconscious mind. It is the master key to
the control of emotions and to operations of the involuntary
(autonomic) nervous system.
– *8 Weeks to Optimum Health*
Andrew Weil, M.D.

You have the power to change, assume responsibility for your self-
care, heal, and be healthier than you have ever been. Several relaxation techniques for stress management are available.

Validation That Relaxation Techniques Do Work

Evidence exists that relaxation methods really do work and could be useful
to you in managing your fibromyalgia and in being well. You may wish to
review the autonomic nervous system in Chapter 4; all stress management
techniques aim to induce a positive parasympathetic state.

In 1996, a National Institutes of Health (NIH) nonfederal, nonadvo-
cate, 12-member panel representing the fields of family medicine, social
medicine, psychiatry, psychology, public health, nursing, and epidemiol-
ogy, along with 23 other experts, concluded that a number of existing well-
defined behavioral and relaxation interventions are effective in treating

chronic pain and insomnia. The NIH panel found strong evidence for the use of relaxation techniques in reducing chronic pain in a variety of medical conditions (NIH Technology Assessment Panel on Integration of Behavioral and Relaxation Approaches Into the Treatment of Chronic Pain and Insomnia. JAMA 1996;276:313–318).

Breathing

Andrew Weil, M.D., is a renowned authority on mind-body interactions. He emphasizes that breathing can exert a strong influence on *mind, body,* and mood. Directing attention to breathing moves you in the direction of relaxation. He says, "The single most effective relaxation technique I know is conscious regulation of breath." He teaches a yogic breathing exercise that can be done in any body position and that he considers a natural tranquilizer for the nervous system. The breathing exercise becomes more effective with repetition and practice (*Natural Health, Natural Medicine,* Boston, New York: Houghton Mifflin Company, 1995).

Breathing also has relevance to *spirit.* This is addressed in the following discussion of the "relaxation response."

The Relaxation Response: A Form of Meditation

The "relaxation response" was initially described by Herbert Benson, M.D., and his colleagues at Harvard Medical School in the early 1970s and most recently in his book, *Timeless Healing: The Power and Biology of Belief* (New York: Scribner, 1996). Margaret A. Caudill, M.D., Ph.D., describes the use of the relaxation response in her book, *Managing Pain Before It Manages You* (New York: The Guilford Press, 1995). The relaxation response can quiet the body's response to stress and can counteract the fight-or-flight response (Chapter 5). However, the fight-or-flight response is automatic, while the relaxation response takes some practice to counteract stress.

Dr. Benson reviewed historical writings of philosophy and religion and concluded that a calming and quieting reflex that can counteract the

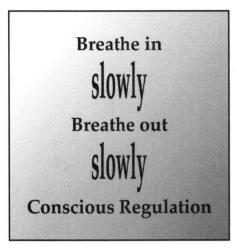

Breathe in

slowly

Breathe out

slowly

Conscious Regulation

fight-or-flight response has been used for centuries through many techniques. Two simple steps are common to all forms of meditation:

- Focusing the mind on a repetitive word, sound, prayer, phrase, or muscular activity, such as breathing.
- Adopting a passive attitude toward the thoughts that go through the head. In other words, everyday thoughts that come to mind should be passively disregarded and attention returned to the repetition.

MindBodySpirit benefits of the relaxation response

Research has shown that practicing and using the relaxation response diminishes the fight-or-flight response. Thus, symptoms resulting from chronic stress are reduced. These beneficial effects of the relaxation response include

- **Immediate benefits** (which occur as the person focuses upon a repetitive word, phrase, breath, or action)   The immediate changes include lowered blood pressure, heart rate, breathing rate, and oxygen consumption (which means that the metabolic rate drops).

- **Long-term benefits** (which occur after practicing for at least a month and persist even when a person is not practicing the relaxation response)   The long-term changes appear to be due to an alteration of the body's response to adrenaline, the stress hormone made by the adrenal gland. The regular practice and use of the relaxation response can result in a reduction in anxiety/depression, functional *MindBodySpirit Symptoms* and *MindBodySpirit Syndromes,* and improvement in the ability to cope with the stresses of life.

- **Spirit**   In Chapter 3, you learned that Harvard research has confirmed that people who elicited the relaxation response experienced a sense of increased spirituality. Spirituality was considered to be the experience of the presence of a power, force, energy, or perception of God. This presence was perceived as close to the person.

Difference between relaxation and relaxation response

Being relaxed and engaging in the relaxation response is not the same unless being relaxed includes both a focus upon a repetitive stimulus and a passive attitude. The relaxation response is not obtained by reading a book, listening to quiet music, sleeping, or relaxing. These activities may be very relaxing, but they are not the same as invoking the relaxation response.

The technique of the relaxation response

Here is the generic technique of the relaxation response that Dr. Benson describes in his book:

Step 1.   Pick a focus word or short phrase that is firmly rooted in your belief system.

Step 2.   Sit quietly in a comfortable position.

Step 3.   Close your eyes.

Step 4.   Relax your muscles.

Step 5.   Breathe slowly and naturally, and as you do, repeat your focus word, phrase, or prayer silently to yourself as you exhale.

Step 6.   Assume a passive attitude. Don't worry about how well you're doing. When other thoughts come to mind, simply say to yourself, "Oh, well," and gently return to the repetition.

Step 7.   Continue for 10 to 20 minutes.

Step 8.   Do not stand immediately. Continue sitting quietly for a minute or so, allowing other thoughts to return. Then open your eyes and sit for another minute before rising.

Step 9.   Practice this technique once or twice daily.

Reprinted with the permission of Scribner, a Division of Simon & Schuster from *Timeless Healing: The Power and Biology of Belief* by Herbert Benson, M.D., with Marg Stark. Copyright 1996 by Herbert Benson, M.D.

The relaxation response can also be done with eyes open and in other body positions, like standing or lying down.

Exercise and the relaxation response

Focused exercise activates the relaxation response. Exercise becomes more efficient as less energy is required to do the physical work. The relaxation response can be elicited during endurance exercise, such as walking or jogging, by paying attention to the cadence of the repetitive movement in the exercise, like the feet hitting the pavement. Unfocused exercise such as listening to a headset radio or watching television while exercising does not invoke the same benefits of the relaxation response.

Exercise

Exercise (Chapters 29 and 30) is beneficial in stress management even without the application of the relaxation response. Exercise is an important component in recovering from fibromyalgia and in living a healthy life.

Yoga

Yoga is a combination of exercise and mental relaxation. It is really a form of moving meditation.

Laughter

Josh Billings, a nineteenth century humorist said, "There ain't much fun in medicine, but there's a heck of a lot of medicine in fun." There is strong scientific evidence that the opposite of the stress response is laughter and that the beneficial changes that occur in the body are real and measurable.

Norman Cousins emphasized this in his book, *Anatomy of an Illness*, (New York: Bantam, Doubleday, Dell, 1991) in which he used humor and laughter to recover from a serious disease. He reported that ten

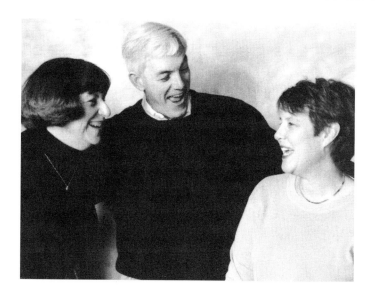

minutes of solid belly laughter would provide him with two hours of pain-free sleep. The popular movie, *Patch Adams* (1998), makes the same point. Duke University has prepared a list of humorous materials available to its patients.

Resources

- The Mind/Body Medical Institute, under the direction of Herbert Benson, M.D., at the Deaconess Hospital in Boston, has a number of relaxation tapes that can be purchased.

  Mind/Body Medical Institute
  110 Francis Street
  Boston, MA 02215
  (617) 632-9525

  Relaxation tapes can be helpful when you are first learning the relaxation response.

- *Managing Pain Before It Manages You,* by Margaret A. Caudill, M.D., Ph.D. (New York: The Guilford Press, 1995) is the book used at

Mind/Body Medical Institute affiliates around the country and can be used by people who are not participating in a formally structured program of pain and symptom management and mind/body medicine.

- *Natural Health, Natural Medicine,* by Andrew Weil, M.D., (Boston, New York: Houghton Mifflin Company, 1995). The breathing technique is presented, along with much advice about stress management and being well.

- Full-text copy of the NIH Technology Assessment Panel on Integration of Behavioral and Relaxation Approaches into the Treatment of Chronic Pain and Insomnia are available. Contact

  NIH Consensus Program Information Center
  PO Box 2577
  Kensington, MD 20891
  (888) NIH-CONSENSUS (644-2667)
  World Wide Web (http://text.nlm.nih.gov/nih/nih.html)

In the next chapter, you will learn how your thoughts can be hurtful or helpful to you.

Chapter 22

Cognitive Behavioral Therapy

Ya Gotta Wanna
– Robert D. Sherer

> Dennis C. Turk, Ph.D., and Justin M. Nash, Ph.D., stress that most
> people do not realize how much their thoughts *(mind)* can affect
> their mood and *body*, including their sensation of pain (*Chronic
> Pain: New Ways to Cope*, in *Mind-Body Medicine: How to Use Your
> Mind for Better Health*, Daniel Goleman, Ph.D., and Joel Gurin
> (eds.), Yonkers, New York: Consumer Reports Books, 1993).

An Example

It is very common for people in chronic pain from fibromyalgia to tell
themselves, "I don't believe that this pain is ever going to get better," or
"I just can't stand this anymore." This self-defeating thinking can actually
aggravate your pain by making it harder to accept the responsibility that
you can control it. Also, the pain gate can be opened, which increases the
pain and discomfort (Chapter 4). Finally, stressful thoughts like these can
cause muscles to tighten up.

Cognitive Behavioral Treatment

Managing chronic pain and symptoms requires the exploration of the relationship of thoughts *(mind)* to *body* symptoms. The source of thoughts
and feelings is the *mind,* which gives meaning to experience, including
symptoms and pain. The *mind* is a "filter" or "lens" through which the
message coming from the *body* passes. The filter or lens can either reduce

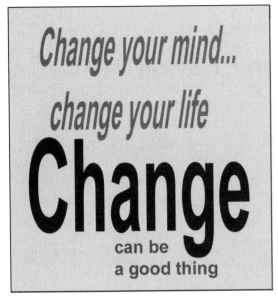

or magnify the intensity of the message. Thus, the experience of pain and symptoms can be lessened or eliminated.

Certain techniques can be learned which allow you to explore how you see the world around you and interpret what happens to you. These techniques are called *cognitive.* The word comes from *cognition,* which means knowing or thinking. Cognitive behavioral therapy is oriented to correcting thinking and thoughts that are "automatic" and counterproductive. An example is changing the unconscious decision to stay in bed instead of going to work when fibromyalgia flares up. In this way, the focus is shifted away from the negative elements of the individual's life.

You can learn these techniques, either by working with a health-care professional, or by using materials such as Dr. Margaret Caudill's book, *Managing Pain Before It Manages You* (New York: The Guilford Press, 1995). Another recent book which we can recommend is *Life Strategies: Doing What Works; Doing What Matters,* by Phillip C. McGraw, Ph.D. (New York: Hyperion, 1999).

Who Should Consider Cognitive Behavioral Treatment?

There are really no guidelines for determining which patients should consider cognitive therapy. But, it would certainly be worth a try if you have emotional distress associated with uncomfortable *body* symptoms (like those with fibromyalgia), are not responding to the measures previously discussed in this book, or have not improved with psychopharmacological drug treatment like the antidepressants (Chapter 23).

Psychotherapy

Even though emotional distress does not cause fibromyalgia, it can make people more vulnerable to stress and make the symptoms worse. Psychological treatments assist people with *MindBodySpirit Symptoms* and *MindBodySpirit Syndromes* to learn to cope with stress and can help control, reduce, or eliminate symptoms. Psychotherapy and counseling can help some people with fibromyalgia by bringing self-understanding and identification of important emotional conditions that can be treated.

The next chapter will show you how antidepressant medications can be used as pain relievers.

Chapter 23

Antidepressant Drugs: Depression and Symptom Relief

> When one door of happiness closes, another opens, but we look so long at the closed door that we do not see the one that has been opened for us.
> – Helen Keller

Antidepressants can be very helpful in chronic pain conditions like fibromyalgia. They can act as pain and symptom relievers operating at the brain level, even in doses lower than needed to treat depression. But if depression is also present, then full doses of antidepressant medication may be necessary.

Pain Control Even without Depression

Antidepressant drugs act as brain analgesics and not just as a treatment for depression. Review the gate-control theory, which discusses how pain can be "blocked" or reduced by the brain (Chapter 4). Antidepressants increase the release of neurotransmitters, chemicals in the brain that cause signals to be sent down the inhibitory pathway. This "closes the gate" in the spinal cord and blocks the transmission of pain signals from the *body* to the *brain.*

Antidepressant drugs can benefit people with chronic pain regardless of whether depression exists. However, these drugs have not been approved formally by the Food and Drug Administration (FDA) for treatment of chronic pain without associated depression. Many people who have chronic pain are also depressed (often only mildly). It can be very difficult for the doctor and patient to determine whether the pain is causing the depression or whether the depression is causing the pain. Fortunately, the successful control of pain with antidepressant drugs does not seem to be dependent upon the presence of depression.

Antidepressant drugs used to treat chronic pain often work in lower doses than are needed to treat depression and other psychological problems. Of course, full doses can be used if the symptoms are associated with depression, not only to treat the depression, but also because depression can lower pain threshold and increase pain sensation.

If Depression Is Present

It is important to treat emotional distress like depression if it does not respond to self-care measures or if severe. You have learned how emotional distress contributes to the symptoms of fibromyalgia through the *Mind-BodySpirit Connection*. Chapter 19 provided information that you can use as a screen for depression. Treating depression may require higher doses of antidepressant drugs than treatment of pain and sleep disturbance.

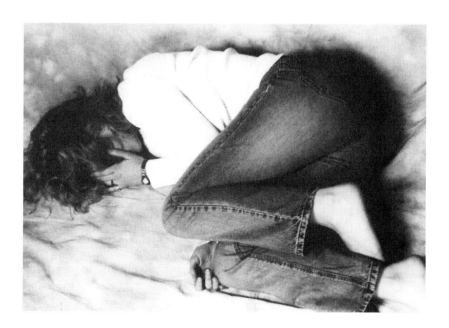

Sleep Enhancement

Sleep disturbance is involved in the causation of fibromyalgia (Chapter 11). Most patients with fibromyalgia experience difficulty in falling asleep, staying asleep, and awakening refreshed. So, they have intensified morning aching and pain.

Many antidepressants are very effective when used to enhance sleep, even in low dosage and when depression is not present. When sleep disturbance is corrected, it results in more restful sleep. As a result, pain is reduced, mood is improved, and energy levels are increased. Some antidepressant drugs are better than others in facilitating sleep, and some may actually interfere with sleep. Your physician will help you select the proper drug.

Prescription sleeping drugs may increase the amount of sleeping time but generally do not improve the quality of sleep. So, they are generally not recommended for treating fibromyalgia.

A Part of a Program of Wellness

The use of antidepressant drugs in the management of fibromyalgia presupposes their use in conjunction with physical exercise, proper diet, weight control, and stress management. Improvement in physical conditioning and in sleep may well result in such improvement that antidepressant medication dosage can be reduced, or even that the drug can be discontinued.

Be Patient: It Takes Time

It can take several weeks for the antidepressants to take effect. If treatment is stopped too soon, then it may appear that the treatment did not work. If you experience side effects, discuss them with your doctor. Most side effects will either diminish or go away completely after several days, or they can be reduced temporarily by lowering the dose. Furthermore, the decision to continue treatment or consider a change of medication can be re-evaluated at an appointment later.

Since everyone is different, trying one or two different antidepressant drugs may be necessary to find the one that is best for you. It is important to assume an active role in trying to get better and deal with the chronic problem. By taking an active role, you will feel in control.

Previous Experience and Concerns

If you have previously taken antidepressants, tell your doctor which drugs you have taken and relate any concerns you might have about this type of treatment. Some people who are reluctant to take antidepressants say that they tried them before (probably for only a very short period of time) and that they either did not help or they produced unpleasant side effects. As a result, they stopped taking the medication.

Some people say they do not want to be controlled by a medicine or to take "mind-altering" drugs. Others are worried that they might become addicted to the treatment. Some are convinced that the problem is not "all in the head" or that family and friends would disapprove.

Discuss your concerns with your doctor because antidepressants can be quite helpful and should be considered, particularly if more conservative treatments are not working. Antidepressant drugs are not addictive.

Three Types of Antidepressant Drugs

It is helpful to classify the antidepressant drugs into three categories: tricyclic antidepressants (TCAs), the selective serotonin reuptake inhibitors (SSRIs), and the atypical antidepressants.

Tricyclic antidepressants

Examples of this class include amitriptyline (Elavil®, Endep®), doxepin (Adapin®, Sinequan®), imipramine (Janimine®, Tofranil®), nortriptyline (Aventyl®, Pamelor®), and desipramine (Norpramin®, Pertofrane®). The tricyclic antidepressant drugs have been the ones most thoroughly studied in the management of chronic pain and symptoms. Furthermore, some can be useful in treating anxiety and helping to bring sleep.

Side effects of the tricyclic antidepressant drugs

The most common side effects of the TCAs are anticholinergic effects (nausea, vomiting, constipation, and abdominal bloating), orthostatic hypotension (low blood pressure, dizziness, weakness, and even fainting when changing from a lying to sitting or standing position), sedation (drowsiness), sexual dysfunction, and weight gain. In adolescents and young adults, TCAs may cause tachycardia (rapid heartbeat) and mild hypertension (high blood pressure). Elderly patients are more sensitive to the anticholinergic effects and may develop delirium (confusion) with high doses or when they are taking other anticholinergic drugs at the same time.

The most dangerous side effect is the causation or aggravation of some of the heart rhythm disturbances. Very rarely, this can be life threatening. The cardiovascular side effects occur most commonly with amitriptyline.

It is usually best to use a selective serotonin reuptake inhibitor (SSRI) if there is a heart conduction problem because of the rare aggravation by the more anticholinergic TCAs (see next section on SSRIs). Withdrawal symptoms of GI upset, dizziness, headache, malaise, increased perspiration, nightmares, and salivation can occasionally occur if the TCA is discontinued abruptly, so the dosage should be tapered when these drugs are stopped after long-term use.

As with any drug, many different side effects can occur. If necessary, it is always safest to check with your doctor if there are any unexplained symptoms that are of concern. Many side effects and symptoms are dose related, meaning that they can be reduced or eliminated by lowering the dose of the TCA.

Specific precautions with the tricyclic antidepressant drugs
- TCAs can interfere with warfarin (anticoagulant therapy).
- TCAs can increase the effects of alcohol and other sedatives.
- TCAs can increase the effects of other anticholinergic drugs.
- Cimetidine (Tagamet® or generic) can increase blood levels of the TCAs and reduce their metabolism as if a higher dose were being taken.
- TCAs can interfere with oral diabetic medication and raise or lower blood sugar levels.

- Avoid becoming pregnant while taking TCAs.
- Use caution when performing potentially dangerous tasks, operating machinery, or driving.
- Use caution if heart disease is present, especially with arrhythmias and/or heart block (mainly with amitriptyline).
- Discontinue TCAs several days before elective surgery.

Practical information about taking the tricyclic antidepressants
The TCAs are not potentially addictive medications. But, if you are taking narcotics, sedatives, or hypnotics, then you should be "weaned" off of them under a doctor's supervision.

The TCA is started in low dosage and is usually taken two to three hours before bedtime so that the drug can cause drowsiness and bring sleep. Also, most of the sedative effect will be gone by morning and there should be minimal "hangover" effect. Some people find they are better off if they take the drug even earlier, and a few find it is better if they take it later or even at bedtime. Some experimentation may be needed to find the right timing. There is at least a one-week to three-week delay in obtaining the maximum sleep and pain relieving benefit for any given dose. This means that a dosage change should not be made too rapidly unless adverse side effects are severe and make it necessary.

Occasionally, patients cannot tolerate even the lowest dose of the TCA because it is either too sedating, causes intolerable side effects, or produces too much of a "hangover" the next day. Should this happen, the tablet can be divided in half with a razor blade. A divided tablet or capsule can leave a bad taste or numb the mouth. This can be avoided by wrapping the half tablet or capsule in a small ball of bread and swallowing it whole so the medication won't contact the tongue or the inside of the mouth. When the proper TCA is found, most patients can expect at least a partial relief from their pain and symptoms.

The selective serotonin reuptake inhibitors (SSRIs)
The SSRIs are a newer class of antidepressant medication that offers an alternative to the traditional tricyclic antidepressant drugs. Medications

in both of these two drug classes are equally effective in treating depression, but the SSRIs are considerably more expensive than the tricyclic antidepressants.

There are now five SSRIs. Fluoxetine (Prozac®) was the first one introduced, followed by paroxetine (Paxil®), sertraline (Zoloft®), fluvoxamine (Luvox®) and citalopram (Celexa®).

The SSRIs have fewer sedating, anticholinergic, and orthostatic side effects and do not cause problems with heart rhythm (refer to previous discussion on TCAs). However, doctors have less experience using the SSRIs than the TCAs in the treatment of chronic pain conditions.

It is best to take the SSRI at bedtime in order to minimize any side effects. Some individuals are very sensitive to these drugs and may respond to even lower doses or to taking the drug every other day. These lower doses may be applicable for the treatment of chronic pain as was described in the previous section on TCAs. In other words, using half of the lowest dosage tablet, a lower dosage in liquid form, or a dose every other day may not only be effective in the treatment of chronic pain, but also in treatment of depression in some patients.

Side effects of the SSRIs

- **Nervousness and jitteriness**   If this occurs, it tends to happen during the first few weeks of treatment but can improve with continued treatment. These effects can be lessened or eliminated by lowering the dose and taking the treatment at bedtime.

- **GI distress with loss of appetite, nausea, or diarrhea**   Taking the drug at bedtime may help, and symptoms often lessen or resolve in time.

- **Headaches**   Headaches can occur or be worsened, which is another reason to take the medication at bedtime.

- **Sexual dysfunction with reduced sexual desire and ability to have an orgasm**   These effects may be lessened or eliminated by dosage reduction, taking the drug every other day, or not taking it for two to three sequential days of the week. For example, if sexual dysfunction is a problem, then the drug is not taken on Thursday, Friday, and Saturday, during which sexual dysfunction resolves, but the beneficial effect is not lost. Citalopram (Celexa®) is alleged to have fewer sexual side effects than the other SSRIs.

- **Insomnia and sleep disturbance**   If there is an SSRI-associated sleep disturbance, then trazodone (Desyrel®) can be helpful as a second drug taken at bedtime (see next section).

Atypical antidepressants

Several of the antidepressant drugs are called atypical because they do not fit into either of the first two categories. These drugs include bupropion (Wellbutrin®), nefazodone (Serzone®), trazodone (Desyrel®), venlafaxine (Effexor®), and mirtazapine (Remeron®). Trazodone is helpful as a hypnotic to assist sleep.

Sexual Side Effects of Antidepressant Drugs

Unfortunately, many of the antidepressant drugs can interfere with sexuality by reducing libido and causing difficulty with achievement of erection and orgasm. Here are the antidepressant drugs that are much less likely to cause a problem: Serzone®, Wellbutrin®, Remeron®, and possibly Celexa® (the newest SSRI).

"Natural" Therapy for Depression

Two nondrug approaches to treating depression include regular aerobic exercise (Chapters 29 and 30) and St. John's wort, which is an herbal preparation (Chapter 40).

Take the next step to emphasize self-care and wellness.

REVIEW OF STEP 4

1. Real physical symptoms of fibromyalgia can be related to harmful stress and emotional distress.

2. Use the self-assessment screens to check for possible problems with alcohol and depression, as well as anxiety, panic, somatoform, and eating disorders.

3. Manage your stress by using the relaxation response technique.

4. Consider cognitive behavioral therapy if your symptoms don't respond to treatment.

5. Antidepressant drugs can be very helpful in the treatment of fibromyalgia, whether depression is present or not.

STEP 5

EMPHASIZING SELF-CARE
AND WELLNESS

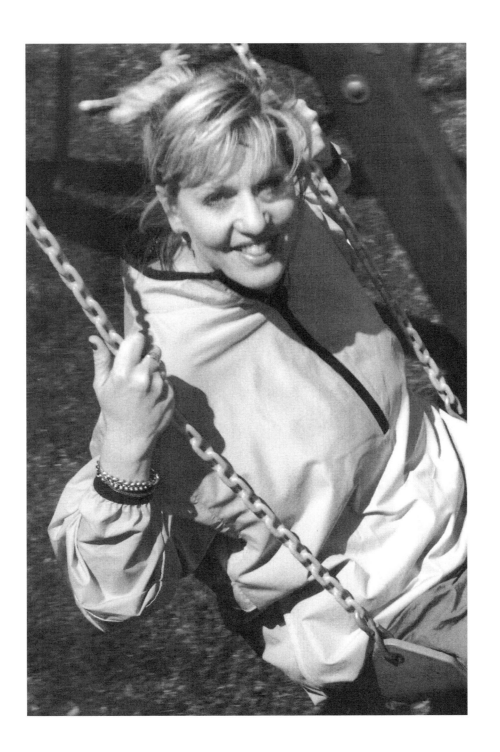

Chapter 24
Healing Is Your Responsibility

Work with your doctor, and with unconventional practitioners
if you so choose, to learn self-care habits. . . . I consider self-care
anything an individual can do, independent of doctors or
healers, to enhance his or her health.
— *Timeless Healing, the Power and Biology of Belief*
Herbert Benson, M.D. (with Marg Stark)

You can heal. You now have a strong awareness of your ability to do
so by understanding the *MindBodySpirit Connection,* accepting responsibility for your health, and making a commitment to self-care.

Understanding the MindBodySpirit Connection

"Knowledge is power," and you have both when you understand the
MindBodySpirit Connection. You know that *mind, body,* and *spirit* are
linked and inseparable. You know how information, including emotion,
is transmitted throughout by chemical messengers called neurotransmitters. And you understand that a biopsychosocialspiritual perspective is
necessary in order to heal. It no longer "works" to think that it's either a
disease or all in the head. You also have a new language that is positive
instead of negative:

- *MindBodySpirit Connection*
- *MindBodySpirit Symptoms*
- *MindBodySpirit Syndromes*
- *MindBodySpirit Healing*

Review the "cause" of fibromyalgia in Chapter 11 and reflect upon what you have learned about your ability to heal in the last two steps. Healing comes from within *you.*

You Are Responsible for Your Health

The model of interaction between patient and doctor is changing so that you, the patient, assume the responsibility for your health in partnership with your doctor and caregiver. In order to do so, you will need accurate and reliable information. Accurate information leads to healing and is often more important than medication.

A healthy diet, weight control, exercise, and stress management are essential for self-care and wellness. Effective treatment of fibromyalgia must include attention to the whole person: the *mind, body,* and *spirit* through the *MindBodySpirit Connection.*

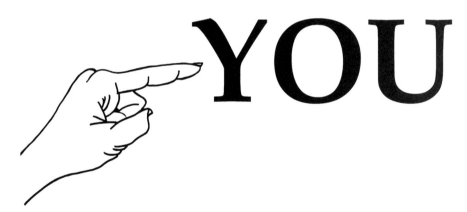

Remember the difference between treatment and healing: treatment originates from the outside, while healing originates from the inside. Treatment of fibromyalgia directed to the *body* without addressing the *mind* and *spirit* may be well intentioned, but it is misguided, ignores self-care and wellness, and does not lead to healing.

Your Control through the MindBodySpirit Connection

Norman Cousins wrote, "In general, anything that restores a sense of control to a patient can be a profound aid to a physician in treating serious illness. That sense of control is more than a mere mood or attitude and may well be a vital pathway between the brain, the endocrine system, and the immune system. The assumed possibility is that it may serve as the basis for what may well be a profound advance in the knowledge of how to confront the challenge of serious illness" (*Head First: The Biology of Hope,* E.P. Dutton: New York, 1989).

You gain power over your illness just by taking a step or steps to be in control. We would like to emphasize that the commitment and decision to take control are just as important as the details of your strategy.

"Use" Fibromyalgia

You are the only one who can do it. It takes commitment and change. Not only can you heal from fibromyalgia, but you can also be healthier than you have ever been.

That's why we said in the Introduction of this book, *You can "use" fibromyalgia to change your life and health.* Turn the negative of your illness into the positive of health and wellness. Heal from fibromyalgia and become healthier than you have ever been before.

Take the steps you need for your self-care. As you do so, maintain awareness of the *MindBodySpirit Connection.*

In the next chapter, you will learn about the importance of sleep in fibromyalgia.

Chapter 25
Sleep

The beginning of health is sleep.
– Irish proverb

Oh Sleep! It is a gentle thing,
Beloved from pole to pole.
– Samuel Taylor Coleridge

For centuries, poets, philosophers, and scientists have studied, analyzed, and commented upon sleep. Several major medical centers have "sleep" laboratories. Television commercials and health stores tout the miraculous powers that mattresses, pillows, and "natural" herbal substances have to produce more restful and restorative sleep. *Proper sleep is particularly important in healing with fibromyalgia and being healthy.*

Questions about Sleep

Many aspects of sleep are not understood.

- What triggers the brain and the body to abandon activity for rest?
- What occurs within the brain as we sleep?
- How do sleep needs and patterns change as we grow older?
- Why do some people need eight to ten hours of sleep, while others seem to function well on as little as four hours?
- Why do some people awaken from sleep feeling restored and full of energy, while others awaken fatigued and groggy?

Stages of Sleep

The "sweet sleep" to which Shakespeare refers in *Othello* is the high quality, restful sleep that we all seek every night. During a typical night's sleep, we journey through different phases of sleep. Researchers now recognize two distinct phases of sleep: REM sleep and non-REM sleep.

REM sleep

REM stands for *rapid eye movement* and is an important phase of the sleep cycle where most dreaming occurs. It typically lasts about 90 minutes, and if REM sleep is disturbed, a person may awaken groggy and without feeling refreshed.

Non-REM sleep

This sleep can be divided into four distinct phases:

Stage 1: Drifting off

The person is awake during this phase, which lasts about 10 minutes. Some begin to experience dreaming here. A loud noise or disturbance during Stage 1 can lead to a "startle" reflex and to reawakening.

Stage 2: Deepening

The separation from consciousness and the awakened state grows. Body metabolism slows, and this phase lasts about 20 minutes.

Stage 3: Increased deepening

The person may be more difficult to awaken during this initial phase of deep sleep, which lasts about 45 minutes.

Stage 4: Deepest, delta wave sleep

This is the deepest sleep which lasts about an hour and which is also known as "slow wave sleep." This refers to slow delta waves recorded on an EEG.

After Stage 4, most people return to Stage 2 before entering REM sleep where most of the dreaming occurs. People continue cycling through these phases of sleep during the night until they awaken naturally or are awakened. Most people will not awaken on their own until they have completed REM sleep. For restful and restorative sleep, it is important that one experience all stages of sleep, particularly Stage 4, where the deepest sleep occurs.

Consequences of Poor Sleep

By contrast, poor sleep habits can contribute to poor health and amplify and enhance the pain and symptoms of fibromyalgia. A scientific study by Moldofsky and Scarisbrick in 1975 showed that sleep deprivation, especially interruption of Stage 4 sleep, produced fibromyalgia symptoms in otherwise healthy adults. Many authorities agree that Stage 4 sleep disturbance is a key factor in causing fibromyalgia (Chapter 11).

Not all people with Stage 4 sleep disorder have fibromyalgia, but virtually all patients with fibromyalgia have Stage 4 sleep disorder (Figure 25.1).

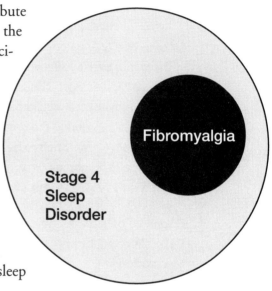

Figure 25.1

Interference with Stage 4 Sleep

Age affects sleep patterns. Young adults spend a large amount of time in Stage 4 sleep. Older adults over age 50 spend less time in Stage 4 sleep. Emotional distress, like anxiety and depression, can interfere with one's ability to fall asleep or cause early awakening so that there is a reduction in the total time spent in Stage 4 sleep. Alcohol and caffeine can also reduce deep sleep time. Many sleeping medications promote loss of consciousness but actually reduce the amount of time spent in deep sleep. Antidepressant drugs are effective in treating the sleep disturbance of fibromyalgia because they increase Stage 4 sleep.

Table 25.1 lists our approach to improving your sleep.

Table 25.1

Approach to Better Sleep

General
Relax for at least one hour before going to bed.
Allow the mind and body to relax (e.g., meditation).
Go to bed only when sleepy.
Get out of bed if you are unable to sleep.
Keep a regular sleep schedule.
Reserve the bed and bedroom for sleep and sex.
Try not to nap during the day.
Avoid heavy meals before bedtime.
Avoid caffeine and alcohol, particularly in the evening.
Get regular exercise, but avoid it just before bedtime (Chapters 29 and 30).
Cognitive behavioral therapy (Chapter 22)
Relaxation techniques (Chapter 21)
Medication
Some prescription or over-the-counter drugs interfere with sleep.
Benzodiazepines
Antidepressants
"Natural" remedies
Sleep study in the laboratory

Benefits of Sleep

Even though many questions remain unanswered, the evidence is clear that a good night's sleep is essential to physical and psychological well being. This is particularly true for those who suffer with fibromyalgia. Sleep has the power to

- Improve mood
- Reduce pain
- Bring calm
- Provide energy
- Sharpen mental alertness
- Increase productivity
- Improve overall health

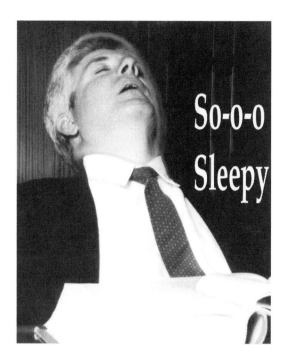

Medication

It can be helpful to check with a doctor or pharmacist to be sure that prescription drugs or over-the-counter medications are not contributing to the sleep problem. Here is a brief discussion of the medications that can be prescribed to help with sleep, which is so important in the treatment of fibromyalgia.

Benzodiazepines

Generally, the use of hypnotic sleep medications like the benzodiazepines should not be the first choice for aiding sleep. If they are used, they should be part of a good sleep hygiene program as previously discussed and used on a short-term or intermittent basis.

Four benzodiazepine drugs—temazepam (Restoril®), flurazepam (Dalmane®), triazolam (Halcion®), and estazolam (ProSom®)—and one non-benzodiazepine zolpidem (Ambien®) are used as hypnotics in the United States. Two other benzodiazepine drugs, lorazepam (Ativan®) and clonazepam (Klonopin®), are also frequently used for this purpose. Note that zolpidem is included here because it activates the benzodiazepine receptor in the brain even though it is not a benzodiazepine.

Antidepressants

Several of the antidepressant drugs (e.g., tricyclics and trazadone) have sedative properties and are useful in the treatment of fibromyalgia to help

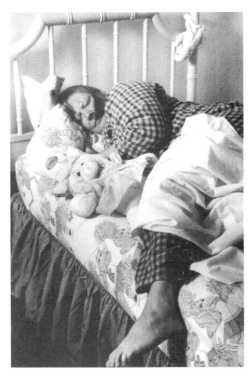

sleep and relieve depression if it is present. Refer to Chapter 23 for more detailed information about antidepressant medications.

"Natural" Remedies

Melatonin

Melatonin is a hormone used by many people as a "natural" sleeping aid, primarily because of advertising hype. Melatonin is sold over-the-counter as a dietary supplement rather than a drug, so the FDA is not involved in quality control or in evaluation of safety and effectiveness.

Melatonin is a hormone. In 1996, the National Institutes of Health held a conference on melatonin and concluded that even though there had been no catastrophic side effects, there was very little information available on long-term safety and usefulness, and there could be occasional side effects. We do not advocate use of this hormone as a solution to managing the sleep disturbance of fibromyalgia.

Valerian

This herb is used throughout the world as a sleeping aid. It is discussed in Chapter 40.

Sleep Study (Polysomnography)

The specialized testing of sleep in which the patient actually sleeps in a laboratory is usually not necessary. The indications for a specialized study of sleep (polysomnography) are somewhat controversial, but they include

- Poor sleep for at least 6 months without an evident cause
- Failure to respond to treatment

- Sleep-related breathing disorder and limb movement disorder. Either can result in continuous arousal movements during sleep that interferes with restful and restorative sleep.
- Restless leg syndrome (RLS). Harvey Moldofsky, M.D., of the University of Toronto, describes this as someone playing soccer all night long. The patient's arms and legs just cannot stay still.
- Periodic limb movement syndrome (PLMS). Dr. Moldofsky says that this may feel like a startling response that you have when you think you have reached the last step going down a flight of stairs and you fling your limbs to catch your balance as you discover that there is one step that remains.

Restless leg syndrome and periodic leg movement syndrome can be treated with a benzodiazepine that has antiseizure properties, such as clonazepam. Tricyclic antidepressant drugs can actually make these conditions worse.

In the next chapter, you will learn about the fundamentals of a healthy diet.

Chapter 26
Healthy Diet

Eat to live and not live to eat.
Wish not so much to live long as to live well.
– from *Poor Richard—An Almanac*
Benjamin Franklin

Committing to a healthy diet is an important step in taking control
and responsibility for your health and recovery from fibromyalgia.

The Importance of a Healthy Diet

Studies now show that around 300,000 people die every year as a result of
diseases related to poor diet or inadequate physical activity. A healthy diet
reduces the risk of developing chronic diseases like heart disease, some
cancers, diabetes, stroke, and osteoporosis. These are the leading causes of
death and disability among Americans. A healthy diet can reduce major
risk factors for chronic diseases like obesity, high blood pressure, and high
blood cholesterol.

This chapter will provide the important and essential nutritional prior-
ities, based upon our experience and sense of the latest science, the latest
government recommendations, and advice from authorities on health and
management of chronic pain such as that associated with fibromyalgia.
Specific menus and recipes will not be given, but the information here
should serve as a guide as you take control by developing your eating plan
for self-care and wellness.

Eating Rules

Whenever possible, try to select either fresh or frozen foods. Margaret A. Caudill, M.D., Ph.D., includes a chapter on nutrition and pain in which she says that "fresh is best" (*Managing Pain Before It Manages You,* New York: The Guilford Press, 1995). Foods prepared by others before they get to our households are more likely to have added salt, sugar, saturated fats, preservatives, and artificial coloring. Furthermore, fiber and nutritional content decrease with increased processing, which is done to give foods a longer shelf life. Processing is also done to satisfy the appetite of the average American consumer who has been eating a diet high in fat and sodium and low in fiber.

It is probably intuitive that you should try to eat in moderation while in a relaxed atmosphere without hurry. This can be easier said than done because of the hectic pace of our lives. Take the time to chew food properly and enjoy the sensations. Proper chewing and eating slowly increase the probability that the digestive system will function well. Frequent, smaller meals spaced through the day may result in less discomfort than eating one or two larger meals.

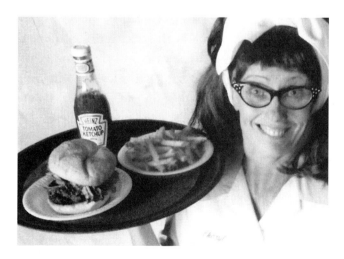

Six Nutritional Issues

Kenneth H. Cooper, M.D., the "Father of Aerobics," explains in his book, *It's Better To Believe,* (Nashville, Thomas Nelson Inc., 1995) that there are four basic nutritional concerns that should govern your grocery shopping and food preparation: fat-cholesterol, fiber, calcium, and supplements. We will add two more, since new information relative to carbohydrate and protein is relevant here. The first five will be discussed in this chapter, and Chapter 27 will address the supplement issue.

- The fat-cholesterol issue
- The carbohydrate issue
- The fiber issue
- The protein issue
- The calcium issue
- The supplement issue, including vitamins, antioxidants, and minerals

The Fat-Cholesterol Issue

Strive to keep the consumption of fats—especially saturated fats—as low as possible. The more saturated fat you consume, the greater the risk of developing high blood cholesterol, heart attack, stroke, circulation problems, and certain types of cancer (like cancer of the colon). Furthermore, there are more calories in a gram of fat (9 calories) than in each gram of protein or carbohydrate (4 calories). Thus, those who eat fat are more likely to have a weight-control problem and become obese.

Fat contains the most calories per serving

Of the three sources of calories in our diet—fat, carbohydrate, and protein—fat is the most nutritionally dense. This means that fat contains the most calories per gram (9), while carbohydrate and protein contain only 4 calories per gram. So eating fat contributes to the problem with weight control and obesity particularly because of the number of calories present in fat. There are over twice as many calories in an equal serving of fat compared to carbohydrate and protein. We will address the restriction of fat caloric intake a little later.

"Bad" fats

You also need to pay attention to the types of fats that you eat and to understand the process used to harden fats called hydrogenation. You particularly want to avoid saturated fats, omega-6 fats, and trans-fats.

Saturated fat
This type of fat raises cholesterol faster than any other type of food. The main sources of saturated fat are whole-fat dairy products, cheeses, red meats, coconut oil, and palm oil.

Polyunsaturated fats (omega-6 fats)
These fats have long been touted as safer than saturated fats. They are found in most vegetable oils (corn, safflower, sesame, soy, and sunflower), margarine, mayonnaise, and commercial salad dressings. But there is a problem with polyunsaturated fat in the form of trans-fatty acids.

Trans-fatty acids from the hydrogenation process
Polyunsaturated omega-6 fats can be chemically changed into trans-fatty acids by a process called hydrogenation, and this unnatural type of fat is a particular risk relative to heart disease. Hydrogenation is a hardening process used to make solid vegetable shortening and which makes potato chips crispier. These unnatural fats are favored by food manufacturers because they oxidize less quickly than does liquid oil, which translates into a longer shelf life.

Avoid foods with these words on the label: "hydrogenated" or "partially hydrogenated." Most trans-fatty acids are hidden from you in commercially baked goods, cookies, crackers, french fries, fried foods, snack foods, margarine, and spreads.

"Good" fats

When possible, substitute olive oil (a monounsaturated omega-9 fat) and fish oil (an omega-3 fat) for "bad" fats. Olive oil is the best all-around oil to use because it contains mainly monounsaturated fat which seems to be better for our bodies than does either saturated or polyunsaturated fat. Populations that rely upon olive oil as their main dietary source of fat have lower rates of both heart disease and cancer than do Americans and most Europeans even though their total fat intake is not that much lower.

Remember that olive oil is still fat and that vegetable oils are the most nutritionally dense source of calories around. Each gram of fat contains 9 calories. So an immoderate intake of olive oil can contribute to obesity.

Fish oil is an omega-3 fat which has beneficial effects. It inhibits the clotting tendency of the blood, reduces the risk of heart attack, improves the serum lipid profile (blood fats), and modifies the production of hormones that control tissue growth and repair, which reduces excessive inflammation and promotes healing. Sources include oily fish from cold, Northern waters (kippers, mackerel, salmon, and sardines) and flaxseed.

Recommendations

Here are our specific recommendations, based upon advice provided by Drs. Cooper, Caudill, Arnot, and *Nutrition and Your Health: Dietary Guidelines for Americans* (Fourth Edition, 1995; U.S. Department of Agriculture and U.S. Department of Health and Human Services). *Dietary Guidelines for Americans* is issued by the federal government to plan federal food programs and formulate nutrition labeling and the government's Food Guide Pyramid. These guidelines are helpful as you seek self-care and wellness. Written for healthy Americans age two years and older about food choices that promote health and prevent disease, the recommendations are updated every five years by a joint committee of the Department of Agriculture and the Department of Health and Human Services.

To meet the recommended Dietary Guidelines for Americans
- Choose a diet with most of the calories from grain products, vegetables, fruits, low-fat milk products, lean meats, fish, poultry, and dry beans.
- Choose fewer calories from fats and sweets.
- Choose a low-fat, low-cholesterol diet.
- Keep your total fat intake to less than 30% of calories daily.

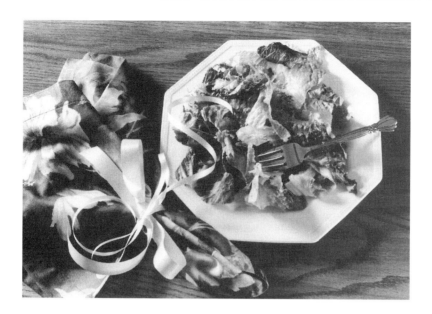

People who need to lose weight or reduce fat for other health reasons (like heart, circulatory problems, and high blood cholesterol) may decide to keep total fat intake below 20% of daily calories. Dr. Cooper recommends that the fat intake be kept below 20% to 25% for the average person older than 30 years of age.

Restrict fat gram calories

You can calculate your daily caloric and fat gram intake. However, you will see that a proper low-fat diet combined with an appropriate exercise program will lead you to an appropriate weight and wellness without actually calculating on a daily basis. Most people, ourselves included, do not like numbers and calculations. Life is already complicated enough!

As recommended by Bob Greene and Oprah Winfrey in their book, *Make the Connection: Ten Steps to a Better Body—and a Better Life,* (New York: Hyperion, 1996), the goal is to reduce the amount of total fat consumed in a day to between 20 and 50 grams. Since humans are all different, you will need to determine what amount works best for you. Some people need to restrict fat more than others do in order to achieve their weight and fitness goals.

You can determine fat grams in food by reading the Nutrition Facts Label on product packages. As an alternative, if you know what percentage of a food is fat, then the fat grams can be calculated. Again, there are 9 calories per gram of fat.

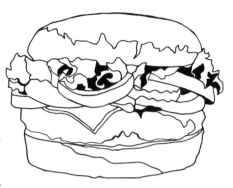

Example of calculating fat grams:

Serving size	= 216 calories, 25% fat
Serving size × 25%	= fat calories
216 × .25 (or 25%)	= 54 fat calories
Fat calories ÷	
9 calories/gram of fat	= fat grams
54 divided by 9	= **6 fat grams**

Limit saturated fat intake to less than 10% of calories daily

Fats contain both saturated and unsaturated (monounsaturated and polyunsaturated) fatty acids. Saturated fat generally comes from animal products and can be identified because it tends to be solid rather than liquid at room temperature. Saturated fat is the more harmful fat and raises blood cholesterol more than the others. Monounsaturated and polyunsaturated fat sources should replace saturated fat sources as often as possible (refer to previous discussion about avoiding hydrogenated and partially hydrogenated fats by substituting olive oil and fish oil).

Limit cholesterol intake to less than 300 mg daily

Cholesterol is not actually a fat; it is a substance found in animal products (mainly eggs, dairy products, and animal fats). The body manufactures all of the cholesterol it needs, but the dietary intake of both fat and cholesterol can contribute to the body's cholesterol production. There are several different types of cholesterol; low-density lipoprotein, or LDL, is the so-called "bad cholesterol."

The Carbohydrate Issue

Carbohydrates serve as the main source of calories and energy. *The Dietary Guidelines for Americans* recommend a diet with most of the calories deriving from grain products, vegetables, fruits, low-fat milk products, and dry beans. However, we feel that you need to be aware that the amount and type of carbohydrates taken may also be important. Considerable controversy surrounds this matter.

Americans eat more fat and <u>relatively</u> more carbohydrate

Studies show Americans eat more grams of fat than ever before, but the percentage of fat eaten has decreased. This means that although Americans have increased the amount of fat eaten, carbohydrate intake has increased even more. So the increase in fat is "diluted" by the intake of excess junk carbohydrate calories. As Robert Arnot, M.D., says in his book, *Dr. Bob Arnot's Revolutionary Weight Control Program* (Little Brown: Boston, 1997), "More fat and more soft carbos produce a one plus one equals ten equation. Neither alone would make us as fat as the combination." Let's take a closer look at this.

Glucose as an energy source

Glucose is the simple sugar that passes from the digestive tract into the bloodstream when carbohydrates are eaten. The term, "blood sugar" is slang for the concentration of glucose in the blood. Almost all carbohydrates are ultimately broken down into glucose, which is the most elemental component. So carbohydrates—from breakfast cereal, pasta, and bread to candy and sugary soft drinks—yield the same result: higher levels of blood sugar. It is obvious that glucose can come from sugar. What is not so obvious is that many of the "complex carbohydrate" low-fat foods composed of large sugar molecules instead of tiny "simple sugars" are rapidly broken down into glucose after they have been digested and absorbed into the bloodstream.

The glucose load and the glycemic index

All of the glucose produced by eating carbohydrates over a day is called the "glucose load." Dr. David Jenkins of the University of Toronto has determined what happens to the blood sugar after foods are eaten on an empty stomach. Each carbohydrate was given a glucose value on a scale ranging from a low of 0 to a high of over 100. This is called the "glycemic index," or "GI." Carbohydrates low on the index like beans, cruciferous vegetables, and high-fiber, low-sugar cereals result in a very small rise in blood sugar after being eaten. These carbohydrates place an insignificant "load" on the system.

By contrast, foods that have a moderate to high glycemic index—like mashed potatoes, white bread, and white pasta—are quickly digested and absorbed, leading to high blood sugar and a high glucose load. These complex carbohydrates may not taste or look sweet, so we tend to eat them without concern. But they are like sugar and result in a high glucose load.

How glucose overload can make you fat

There is some evidence that part of the problem with carbohydrates and obesity is related to insulin. Insulin is the hormone that moves glucose into fat cells. The higher the glucose load, the more insulin is released. The explanation is more complicated than this, and some controversy remains. Let's look at how the contemporary diets seem to work. Carbohydrates may be the key.

How different diets achieve weight loss

Dr. Arnot has pointed out that diets that appear to be very different—like those of Dr. Robert Atkins, Dr. Barry Sears, and Dr. Dean Ornish—succeed because they all reduce the glucose load in different ways. Dr. Atkins drops the glucose load by virtually eliminating all carbohydrates from his diet. Dr. Barry Sears drops carbohydrates in the diet from 60 to 40 percent, increases protein to 30 percent, and fat to 30 percent. Dr. Ornish drops the carbohydrate load by recommending unrefined carbohydrates. These carbohydrates have a lower glycemic index so that the glucose load is reduced. Also, the total amount of carbohydrate intake is lowered because these unrefined carbohydrates are so filling.

Dropping the glucose load

Here is how you can reduce your glucose load. It is not as difficult as you might think.

- Eat low-glucose carbohydrates because they are filling and have a small effect on glucose load. Resources are available that list these low-glucose carbohydrates, including books by Doctors Arnot and Sears, but these foods are mainly beans of all types, certain grains (rice bran, barley, bran, mixed grains), certain fruits (e.g., cherries, plums, grapefruit, fresh peaches, dried apricots, apples, grapes, and oranges), and certain vegetables (dried peas, chickpeas, lentils, tomato). Note that white flour pasta has a medium glycemic index, while whole wheat pastas are in the low-glycemic index category because of less refined flour and more fiber. It is also better to eat whole wheat breads rather than white bread for the same reason.
- Use more vegetable fat to replace moderate and high glycemic index carbohydrates (see preceding discussion on fats).
- Eat more protein to replace moderate and high glycemic index carbohydrates, because insulin levels rise very little. Protein helps to reduce hunger and energize the brain.
- Eat foods with more fiber (see later discussion).

The Fiber Issue

Fiber, also called roughage or bulk, is a type of carbohydrate and is a very important part of a healthy diet for most people. This is why the government guidelines recommend the following:

> **Most people should strive for a daily fiber intake of from 20 to 35 grams per day.**
> *(Nutrition and Your Health: Dietary Guidelines for Americans)*

Definition of fiber

Fiber is found in the cell walls of plant foods, such as whole-grain breads and cereals, beans and peas, and other fruits and vegetables. Fiber cannot be digested or absorbed into our bodies, so it does not provide calories, vitamins, or minerals. Several different types of fiber with different chemical structures and ability to dissolve in water have been identified. It is useful to think of fiber as soluble and insoluble, and both types of fiber are important for healthy digestive function.

Soluble fiber

Soluble fiber disperses well in water and liquid and forms a soft gel in the digestive tract. It is not broken down until it reaches the colon, where its digestion and fermentation cause the production of gas. Examples of soluble fiber are oats, beans, peas, and many types of fruit.

Insoluble fiber

This type of fiber does not disperse in water and liquid and undergoes only minimal change as it passes through the digestive tract. Examples of insoluble fiber include wheat bran, whole-grain breads, and many vegetables.

Benefits of fiber

There are multiple benefits of fiber. Here are the most important ones.

Digestive system

Fiber is necessary to promote normal peristalsis, the wavelike muscular contractions that move the food along the intestinal tract. As fiber passes along, it absorbs water, which softens and bulks up the stool. Higher stool bulk results in softer and larger stools for most people and eases the elimination of the stool. More bulk means that pressure in the colon is actually reduced. The colon does not have to contract as strongly to propel the stool content along. This is important for many people who have constipation, irritable bowel syndrome, diverticulosis, and/or hemorrhoids.

Perineal hygiene can be improved with fiber because cleansing following bowel movements is easier. Some people with diarrhea benefit from increased fiber intake because the stool may become more solid as the fiber absorbs water from it.

Evidence now suggests that increasing dietary fiber may reduce the risk of developing colon polyps and cancer; however, a recent study published in the New England Journal of Medicine called this into question.

Cholesterol and heart disease

There is strong evidence that fiber (especially soluble) can lower blood cholesterol and may reduce the risk of heart disease (see following discussion on psyllium). There is some question as to which type of fiber is optimal and exactly who should take fiber for this purpose. The best approach is to combine a low-fat, high-fiber diet to prevent coronary heart disease. The effect of dietary and supplemental fiber on blood cholesterol levels and atherosclerosis is the subject of considerable research.

How much fiber should I take?

The United States has one of the lowest dietary fiber intakes per capita in the world. The average American only takes in 13 grams of fiber per day. By contrast, Africans take in an average of 60 grams of fiber per day. We recommend keeping two goals in *mind* for your *body*.

1. **Amount of fiber**   Health experts now recommend increasing dietary intake to 20 to 35 grams per day. For most people, this means at least doubling the daily fiber intake. Some people with constipation benefit by taking in even more fiber than the recommended amounts.

2. **Good bowel function**   The normal bowel pattern in the United States is from three bowel movements per day to three bowel movements per week. This means that fiber intake should be adequate to achieve
    - Three or more soft bowel movements per week
    - Comfortable passage of soft stool without undue straining
    - Avoidance of harsh stimulant laxatives

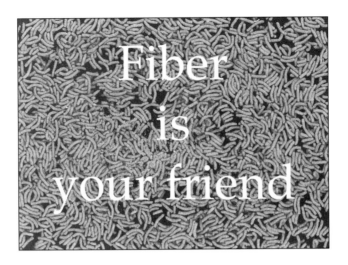

Dr. Salt's partner, Eugene May, M.D., always advises his patients to eat enough fiber so that their bowel movements were "totally tubular and the diameter of a quarter."

How to increase dietary fiber

You can easily increase dietary fiber by eating bran-containing cereals. However, it is important to read labels carefully because many products claiming to be rich in bran and fiber are actually not. Look for cereals that provide 4 to 5 grams per serving.

Increase consumption of fruits and vegetables. For example, add dates, figs, or prunes to the serving of cereal in the morning. Another good source of fiber is cooked beans of all types. They provide approximately 4 to 5 grams of fiber per half-cup serving.

Finally, note that white flour is an extremely poor source of fiber. If you consume fewer products made from white flour and more whole-grain foods of all types along with more fruits and vegetables, you will be successful in increasing dietary fiber.

Add fiber gradually

It is usually best to gradually increase fiber intake over the course of several weeks to reduce the chance of developing "gas," cramping, bloating, and flatulence. Most people find that the symptoms caused by eating more dietary fiber gradually decline over the ensuing one to two months. Furthermore, the relief from constipation or diarrhea is an acceptable trade-off.

Drink adequate amounts of water and fluids

It is important to take plenty of water and fluids when dietary fiber is increased. Try to drink six to eight 8-ounce glasses of fluid each day.

Fiber supplements

It can be difficult to meet the recommended fiber intake of 20 to 35 grams per day through your diet. If this is the case, consider utilizing dietary fiber supplements. Several products are available.

Psyllium   Psyllium is a soluble fiber derived from the husks of psyllium seeds. Clinical trials have confirmed that psyllium lowers cholesterol levels. The Food and Drug Administration has recently approved psyllium with the statement that it may reduce the risk of heart disease when used as a dietary fiber supplement, as part of a diet low in saturated fat and cholesterol, and when taken in a dosage of at least 7 grams per day. All soluble fibers have not been shown to offer these benefits.

Psyllium is the main ingredient of many safe commercially available bulk products such as Fiberall®, Hydrocil®, Konsyl®, Metamucil®, and Perdiem®. Psyllium is generically available and powdered psyllium seed husks can be purchased at a health food store.

Methylcellulose   Methylcellulose is a semisynthetic soluble fiber that does not undergo bacterial fermentation and breakdown. This may result in fewer problems with "gas" and flatulence. Methylcellulose is available as Citrucel®.

Calcium polycarbophil   Calcium polycarbophil is a synthetic fiber that is not fermented and broken down by bacteria. It acts like an insoluble fiber. Commercially available products include Equalactin®, FiberCon®, and Mitrolan®.

If gas and flatulence develop

Remember to introduce fiber gradually, as was discussed earlier. Try to remain optimistic that the symptoms may well diminish or disappear over the following month. Some people have a significant problem with abdominal bloating and flatulence when they increase the fiber content of the diet and do not seem to be able to adjust to the change. They may have an increased sensitivity to what is happening in the digestive tract, mediated through the *MindBodySpirit Connection.*

The gas released by the breakdown and fermentation of the complex carbohydrates of fiber causes distention of the colon that is perceived as discomfort, bloating, and pain. Furthermore, some people are more likely to produce gas than are others. If bran causes gas and flatulence, try reducing intake and concentrate on eating more whole grains, fruits, and vegetables. You can also try fiber supplements, but some products can be better tolerated than others.

The Protein Issue

Protein has a long reputation as the foundation for weight reduction diets. The benefits of protein are that it is a better hunger killer than either fat or carbohydrate, it activates the *mind,* and it serves as a carbohydrate substitute that reduces glucose load.

There is controversy on how much protein should be consumed each day. Many of the contemporary diets recommend nearly tripling the percent of protein in the diet, from 12 percent to 30 percent.

Recent federal guidelines from the FDA Center for Food Safety and Applied Nutrition recommend that women who are 51 years of age and older should consume at least 50 grams of protein each day. Furthermore, new research has shown that adequate amounts of protein reduce the risk of hip fracture in aging women (*American Journal of Clinical Nutrition* 1999;69:147–152).

We recommend that protein intake be 20 to 25 percent of the total caloric intake during the period that you are striving for weight loss. Recommended protein intake also depends upon your level of activity, and needs increase with increasing exercise, particularly resistance training (Chapter 30). Dr. Arnot's book, *Dr. Bob Arnot's Revolutionary Weight Control Program,* has a table recommending protein intake in grams based upon weight and level of exercise activity (Little, Brown and Company: Boston, 1997). He recommends what he calls hard proteins that are low in fats and carbohydrates. This includes hard beans and hard dairy (skim milk, low-fat yogurt without added sugar, egg whites, whey protein, and low-fat cottage cheese).

The Calcium Issue

Calcium plays an important role in building and maintaining bone. It is an important part of a dietary plan; however, national surveys confirm that many Americans do not consume adequate calcium. When calcium intake is inadequate, calcium is removed from the bones in order to maintain normal blood levels.

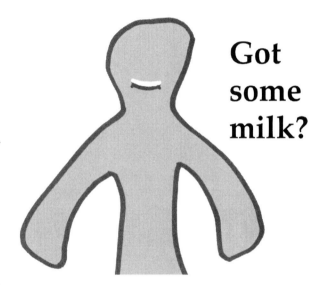

Osteoporosis, the weakening of the skeleton from loss of bone, occurs with increasing age and is a greater problem for women than for men. Twenty-five million Americans are afflicted and 1.5 million bone fractures occur every year as a result. Prevention of osteoporosis is the best strategy because it usually progresses silently until a fracture occurs. Adequate calcium intake is an important part of reducing risk of developing osteoporosis.

There may be other benefits to adequate calcium intake. Recent research has shown a beneficial effect of calcium in reducing symptoms of Premenstrual Tension Syndrome (PMS) and in reducing the risk of developing colon polyps and cancer.

Table 26.1 lists the calcium requirements from the National Institutes of Health Consensus Panel. These requirements can be met through foods, supplements, or a combination of both. The main foods that are calcium-rich are dairy products (milk, cheese, and yogurt). One glass of milk provides 250 mg of calcium. Other sources of calcium include broccoli, kale, mustard and collard greens, tofu, sardines, and salmon.

Table 26.1

Optimal Calcium Requirements

Group	Optimal Daily Intake (in mg of calcium)
Infants	
Birth–6 months	400
6 months–1 year	600
Children	
1–5 years	800
6–10 years	800–1,200
Adolescents/Young Adults	
11–24 years	1,200–1,500
Men	
25–65 years	1,000
Over 65 years	1,500
Women	
25–50 years	1,000
Over 50 years (postmenopausal)	
On estrogens	1,000
Not on estrogens	1,500
Over 65 years	1,500
Pregnant and nursing	1,200–1,500

From National Institutes of Health Consensus Panel, Optimal Calcium Intake, 1994

Multiple calcium supplements are available to ensure adequate intake of 1000 to 1500 mg per day. It is best to take divided doses, with no more than 500 to 600 mg of elemental calcium at one time, and preferably with meals. Calcium carbonate has a high calcium content and low cost. Examples are Caltrate® 600 (600 mg), Tums® (200 mg), and Tums-EX® (300 mg). Generic calcium carbonate is available, but this form of calcium can cause bloating and constipation.

If these side effects occur, if stomach acid levels are low, or if kidney stones are a problem, then calcium citrate can be used (calcium can be taken even if kidney stones are a problem, but it is best to check with a doctor because urine tests may be needed). Examples of calcium citrate are Citracal® (200 mg) and Citracal® Liquitab® (500 mg). Generic calcium citrate is available.

For information about osteoporosis

If you would like to know more about osteoporosis, contact the

National Osteoporosis Foundation
1150 17th Street NW, Suite 500 • Washington, DC 20036-4603
(202) 223-2226 • http://www.nof.org

The next chapter discusses supplements, antioxidants, vitamins, and minerals.

Chapter 27

Supplements, Vitamins, Antioxidants, and Minerals

Many health food stores might better be called pill stores, given how little food they stock in relation to all the vitamins and supplements. Claims made for these products are extravagant. If they were all true, we could forget about proper diet, exercise, relaxation, and all other preventive strategies and just take pills.
– *Natural Health, Natural Medicine*
Andrew Weil, M.D.

Geoffrey Cowley has observed that Americans spend $6 billion every year on nutritional supplements, which includes vitamins and minerals ("Herbal Warning," *Newsweek,* May 6, 1996). Sales are increasing by 20% every year.

Multivitamins

Most adults who are able and willing to eat a balanced diet probably do not need vitamin and mineral supplements. Exceptions are

- Pregnant women who need supplementary iron and folic acid
- People who are on low-calorie diets long term
- People who are recovering from surgery or serious illness whose ability to eat has been altered
- Women who need calcium and vitamin D supplementation to prevent osteoporosis
- The elderly who do not have an interest in eating

It is perfectly safe to take a good multivitamin on a regular basis, and many different brands are available. Many companies allege that natural vitamins are better than the synthetic versions and charge more money; however, there is no evidence that natural vitamins are superior to synthetic vitamins.

Antioxidants

It is now estimated that 40% of the population of the United States is taking antioxidant vitamins and vitamin supplements. This is a result of many scientific and popular press reports of benefits. The chemical reactions within the cells of the body that require oxygen create what are called *free radicals*. These free radicals are highly unstable molecules that are normal products of these reactions. Exposure to cigarette smoke and other pollutants in the environment also brings about oxidation and the release of free radicals. Free radicals not only can damage your cell membranes, but they also can cause cancer and heart disease.

The antioxidants are vitamin A, beta-carotene, vitamin E, ascorbic acid (vitamin C), and the trace mineral selenium. There is now some evidence that the antioxidant vitamins can block the harmful effects of free radicals before damage of the cells occurs. Population studies and small clinical trials have shown that there tends to be lower rates of cancer and heart disease in populations eating foods high in these vitamins.

Expert opinion remains divided about whether taking antioxidant vitamins in dosages higher than the recommended RDA confers additional benefits.

At this time, the most reasonable advice is to eat fruits and vegetables that are rich in these antioxidant vitamins (sweet potatoes, spinach, carrots, broccoli, cantaloupe, and citrus fruits). It should be an individual decision whether to take antioxidant vitamin supplements. There may be some risk to taking megadoses of vitamins. If you decide to take antioxidant vitamins, here are some recommendations.

Vitamin A

Women of child-bearing potential, people with liver disease, and those who consume alcohol heavily should avoid vitamin A. Most cases of vitamin A toxic reactions reported each year in the United States involve doses greater than 100,000 IU (international units) per day. Use beta-carotene instead, or take less than 50,000 IU of vitamin A per day. The safest range would be 5000 to 10,000 IU per day, which is the dosage found in most multivitamins.

Beta carotene

Beta carotene is the water-soluble precursor of vitamin A. It has not been reported to be associated with harmful effects in doses of 30 to 180 mg per day when taken for as long as 15 years. Thus, it seems to be very safe, even at high doses and prolonged exposure. The usual dose is 15 mg, or 25,000 IU per day. If doses larger than 50,000 IU per day are taken, the skin can turn an orange color that is first noted on the palms of the hands. The color disappears if the dosage is reduced.

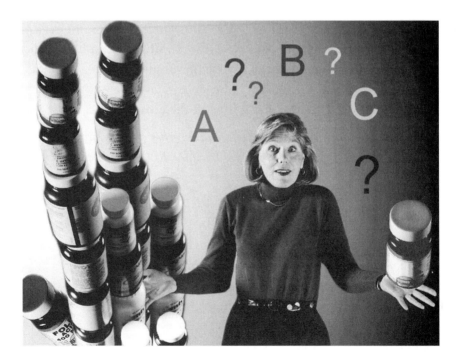

Vitamin E

Vitamin E appears to be safe even at doses as high as 3200 IU per day, but people who take anticoagulant drugs to thin the blood should avoid taking vitamin E unless they discuss it with their doctor. The usual dose is 400 to 800 IU per day.

Vitamin C

Vitamin C is safe at doses less than 4 grams per day, aside from increased crystal formation in the urine and rare kidney stone formation in patients with diminished kidney function or chronic kidney disease. Vitamin C can interfere with many laboratory tests, so you should inform your physician if you are taking it. In high doses, vitamin C can cause diarrhea and flatulence. The usual dosage ranges from 1 gram twice a day to 2 grams three times a day.

Selenium

Selenium is a trace mineral that has recently been shown to have anti-cancer effects. The dose is 100 to 300 micrograms per day.

Vitamin D

Vitamin D is needed to reduce the age-related decrease in calcium absorption. Exposure to sunlight converts vitamin D precursors in the skin to vitamin D, and daily exposure to 20 minutes of sunlight is sufficient to meet vitamin D needs. Nevertheless, many people should avoid sunlight. The recommended daily dose of vitamin D is 400 to 800 international units (IU). This can be obtained in a good multivitamin, and some calcium supplements contain vitamin D. Refer to the previous chapter for a discussion of the importance of adequate calcium intake.

Dietary Supplements

A food supplement is any food substance or mixture of substances taken in place of, or in addition to, food. The most commonly used food supplements are vitamin and mineral pills. Products cannot be marketed with therapeutic claims until shown to be safe and effective by the FDA. However, in 1994, Congress passed the Dietary Supplement Health and Education Act (DSHEA). This classifies vitamins, minerals, and herbs as food supplements instead of drugs, which reduces the Food and Drug Administration's control over them.

Many nutritional products are called dietary supplements even though their use is intended for the prevention or treatment of a health problem. The product label does not include the intended uses. Instead, the intended uses are communicated to stores and the public through books, pamphlets, and word-of-mouth advertisement. The people who promote these products call them supplements while hoping that they will be considered foods rather than drugs in order to be exempt from laws that regulate the sale of drugs.

Many promoters encourage the use of food supplements, claiming that

- It is difficult to obtain necessary vitamins and minerals from regular foods.
- Vitamin and mineral deficiencies are common.
- Most diseases are caused by inadequate diet.
- Most diseases can be prevented by nutritional supplementation.

These concepts are generally not true, and eating according to recommended guidelines is all that is necessary for most adults.

In the next chapter, you will learn what you need to know about weight.

Chapter 28
Weight

By any standard, it's alarming (referring to obesity).
– Arthur Frank, M.D.
(Medical Director, George Washington
University Obesity Management Program)

> There is a national epidemic of obesity. Not only are Americans getting fatter, but also an increasing number are becoming obese.

The "Size" of the Problem

For the first time, more Americans are overweight than are a healthy weight; 55 percent of the adult population of the United States are considered overweight or obese. Obesity is the second leading cause of preventable death in the United States (smoking is number one). The annual death toll from obesity is estimated at 300,000.

A New Definition of Overweight and Obesity

The National Institutes of Health has announced a new definition of overweight and obesity based upon a calculation called the body mass index or BMI. It relates body weight and height and is closely linked to a person's body fat.

You can determine your BMI with a calculator, an example of which is found at the following internet link:

www.nhlbisupport.com/bmi (National Heart, Lung, and Blood Institute)

There are two other ways to determine the body mass index (BMI). One way is to divide body weight by height squared as follows. A second way is to use a table to determine body mass index (see Table 28.1).

Step 1. Multiply weight in pounds by 704.5.

Step 2. Multiply height in inches by height in inches (this is the square of the height in inches).

Step 3. Divide the answer in Step 1 by the answer in Step 2 to calculate the body mass index (BMI).

Table 28.1

Body Mass Index Chart

Height (inches)	19	20	21	22	23	24	25	26	27	28	29	30	31	32	33	34	35	36
								Body Weight (pounds)										
58	91	96	100	105	110	115	119	124	129	134	138	143	148	153	158	162	167	172
59	94	99	104	109	114	119	124	128	133	138	143	148	153	158	163	168	173	178
60	97	102	107	112	118	123	128	133	138	143	148	153	158	163	168	174	179	184
61	100	106	111	116	122	127	132	137	143	148	153	158	164	169	174	180	185	190
62	104	109	115	120	126	131	136	142	147	153	158	164	169	175	180	186	191	196
63	107	113	118	124	130	135	141	146	152	158	163	169	175	180	186	191	197	203
64	110	116	122	128	134	140	145	151	157	163	169	174	180	186	192	197	204	209
65	114	120	126	132	138	144	150	156	162	168	174	180	186	192	198	204	210	216
66	118	124	130	136	142	148	155	161	167	173	179	186	192	198	204	210	216	223
67	121	127	134	140	146	153	159	166	172	178	185	191	198	204	211	217	223	230
68	125	131	138	144	151	158	164	171	177	184	190	197	203	210	216	223	230	236
69	128	135	142	149	155	162	169	176	182	189	196	203	209	216	223	230	236	243
70	132	139	146	153	160	167	174	181	188	195	202	209	216	222	229	236	243	250
71	136	143	150	157	165	172	179	186	193	200	208	215	222	229	236	243	250	257
72	140	147	154	162	169	177	184	191	199	206	213	221	228	235	242	250	258	265
73	144	151	159	166	174	182	189	197	204	212	219	227	235	242	250	257	265	272
74	148	155	163	171	179	186	194	202	210	218	225	233	241	249	256	264	272	280
75	152	160	168	176	184	192	200	208	216	224	232	240	248	256	264	272	279	287
76	156	164	172	180	189	197	205	213	221	230	238	246	254	263	271	279	287	295

To use this table, find the appropriate height in the left-hand column. Move across to a given weight. The number at the top of the column is the BMI at that height and weight. Pounds have been rounded off.

Example:

140 pound woman with a height of 5 feet 5 inches (65 inches)

Step 1. Multiply weight in pounds by 704.5.
$140 \times 704.5 = 98{,}630$

Step 2. Multiply height in inches by height in inches.
$65 \times 65 = 4225$

Step 3. Divide the answer in Step 1 by the answer in Step 2.
$98{,}630 \div 4225 = 23$ (Body Mass Index)

Table 28.1 *(continued)*

Body Mass Index Chart

Height (inches)	37	38	39	40	41	42	43	44	45	46	47	48	49	50	51	52	53	54
								Body Weight (pounds)										
58	177	181	186	191	196	201	205	210	215	220	224	229	234	239	244	248	253	258
59	183	188	193	198	203	208	212	217	222	227	232	237	242	247	252	257	262	267
60	189	194	199	204	209	215	220	225	230	235	240	245	250	255	261	266	271	276
61	195	201	206	211	217	222	227	232	238	243	248	254	259	264	269	275	280	285
62	202	207	213	218	224	229	235	240	246	251	256	262	267	273	278	284	289	295
63	208	214	220	225	231	237	242	248	254	259	265	270	278	282	287	293	299	304
64	215	221	227	232	238	244	250	256	262	267	273	279	285	291	296	302	308	314
65	222	228	234	240	246	252	258	264	270	276	282	288	294	300	306	312	318	324
66	229	235	241	247	253	260	266	272	278	284	291	297	303	309	315	322	328	334
67	236	242	249	255	261	268	274	280	287	293	299	306	312	319	325	331	338	344
68	243	249	256	262	269	276	282	289	295	302	308	315	322	328	335	341	348	354
69	250	257	263	270	277	284	291	297	304	311	318	324	331	338	345	351	358	365
70	257	264	271	278	285	292	299	306	313	320	327	334	341	348	355	362	369	376
71	265	272	279	286	293	301	308	315	322	329	338	343	351	358	365	372	379	386
72	272	279	287	294	302	309	316	324	331	338	346	353	361	368	375	383	390	397
73	280	288	295	302	310	318	325	333	340	348	355	363	371	378	386	393	401	408
74	287	295	303	311	319	326	334	342	350	358	365	373	381	389	396	404	412	420
75	295	303	311	319	327	335	343	351	359	367	375	383	391	399	407	415	423	431
76	304	312	320	328	336	344	353	361	369	377	385	394	402	410	418	426	435	443

Meaning of the Body Mass Index

A BMI over 25 is considered overweight. Obesity is defined as a BMI of 31.1 or higher for males and 32.3 or higher for females.

Table 28.2 relates the BMI and weight-related health risks, which are listed in the next section.

Table 28.2

Body Mass Index and Weight-Related Health Risk*

Body Mass Index (BMI)	Weight-Related Risk
< 25	Minimal risk
25–27	Low risk
27–30	Moderate risk
30–35	High risk
35–40	Very high risk
> 40	Extremely high risk

* Risk may be even greater if a person has a medical condition or family history of certain diseases such as heart disease and/or diabetes.

Why Should People Worry about Weight?

Many Americans gain weight as they age. It is estimated that the average person gains at least one pound of fat and loses one-half pound of muscle each year, beginning at age 20, unless he (she) changes his (her) lifestyle. There is a growing awareness that any amount of excess body fat is a potential health risk for

- Coronary heart disease and heart attack
- Hypertension
- Stroke
- Diabetes
- Gall bladder disease
- Osteoarthritis
- Sleep apnea

- Respiratory problems
- Certain cancers, especially of the breast and endometrium (uterus)

Obesity is expensive, too. The National Institutes of Health estimates that obesity-related disease costs the nation approximately $100 billion each year.

The Purpose of Body Fat

It is actually necessary to have a certain amount of body fat in order to live. Body fat is simply stored energy (or food), and do we humans have an enormous capacity to store it! In ancient times, this storage served as a survival mechanism when food was scarce. In modern times, food has become plentiful in the developed countries. Food is abundant and much of it is loaded with calories.

The Waistline: Location of Body Fat and Health Risk

The location of body fat is also an important matter in health risks for adults. Excess fat in the stomach area (abdomen) is a greater health risk than excess fat in the hips and thighs. In other words, it is a greater risk to look like an apple than a pear.

The BMI is not a perfect measure of fatness. A fit muscular person with low percentage of body fat could end up with the same BMI as someone who is really fat. So the new guidelines also call for the measurement of the waistline. Fat that accumulates around the belly is the most serious threat to health, and the guidelines say that those with a BMI of 25 to 35 face an increased risk of developing serious health problem if

- Waist measurement > 35 inches for women
- Waist measurement > 40 inches for men

Even if your BMI falls into the low-risk range of 21 to 25, carrying too much weight around the middle places you at greater risk than someone whose fat is collected on the hips and thighs. Likewise, people with an acceptable BMI who have gained weight as adults are at greater risk than those who have maintained their college weight.

The waist-to-hip measurement (measure the waist in inches and the hips at the widest point across the buttocks) is also useful. An individual is considered overweight if the ratio is greater than 0.95 for men and greater than 0.80 for women.

How Much Body Fat Is Healthy?

Fat is stored throughout the body. Approximately 50 percent is located just underneath the skin in the subcutaneous tissue, while another 40 percent is marbled inside of the muscles. The remaining 10 percent is located around and in the main organs of the body.

It is not possible to reduce the body fat percentage to below 3% and remain healthy and live. Levels of fat in this range are only seen in some very highly conditioned athletes. However, there are some differences of opinion about how much body fat is ideal. Table 28.3 lists recommendations from four contemporary experts.

Table 28.3		
Ideal Body Fat for Men and Women		
Authority	**Men**	**Women**
Ellington Darden, Ph.D.	Less than 13%	Less than 18%
Kenneth Cooper, M.D.	15–19%	12–22% (never less than 12%)
Covert Bailey	15% = Ideal	22% = Ideal
Bob Greene	8–15%	15–25%

Ellington Darden, Ph.D., *Living Longer Stronger,* (New York: Perigree, 1995); *Body Defining,* (Chicago: Contemporary Books Inc., 1996).

Kenneth Cooper, M.D., *It's Better to Believe,* (Nashville, TN: Thomas Nelson Inc., 1995).

Covert Bailey, *Smart Exercise: Burning Fat, Getting Fit,* (Boston: Houghton Mifflin Company, 1994).

Bob Greene and Oprah Winfrey, *Make the Connection: Ten Steps to a Better Body—and a Better Life,* (New York: Hyperion, 1996).

Note that it is normal and expected that women have more fat than do men by about 7% to 8%. Particularly for women, body fat should not drop below 12% because of an increased risk of amenorrhea (cessation of menstrual periods) and other health problems.

Measuring Body Fat

The percentage of body fat can be determined most accurately by underwater weighing; however, this method is inconvenient, expensive, and not readily available. The most practical method is by use of skin-fold measurements: "the pinch test."

The thickness of the fat beneath the skin is a fairly good reflection of the percentage of total body fat. The YMCA, a fitness center, or a health club will have the capability of providing measurements using a skin-fold caliper to determine the thickness of the folds of skin and fat from certain parts of the body. Plastic skin-fold calipers can be purchased for about $10 to $12 from sporting goods stores and sports and fitness magazines.

Having provided this information about body fat percentage, we agree with Bob Greene and do not recommend having your body fat measured unless you are very

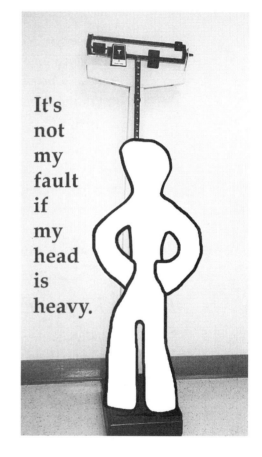

interested or feel that you need the information for motivation. It is difficult to get reproducible results with the pinch test, which is best done by a person skilled in the technique. Furthermore, if you commit to a good program of eating and exercise, you will reduce your body fat and get healthy results, no matter what the numbers show!

What to Do about Excess Weight

Current studies show that even a modest amount of weight loss is beneficial for obese people, especially if other medical problems, such as hypertension, diabetes, or elevated levels of cholesterol, are present.

Federal guidelines regarding nutrition and health are updated every five years. They recommend that people

> **Maintain weight in a single healthy range instead of allowing weight to creep up over the years.**
> (*Nutrition and Your Health: Dietary Guidelines for Americans*
> Fourth Edition, 1995; U.S. Department of Agriculture and
> U.S. Department of Health and Human Services)

The guidelines caution against crash weight loss and suggest slow and steady loss of weight of about ½ to 1 pound per week for those who need to lose weight, through a combination of exercise and healthy eating. Weight reduction of even 5% to 10% of body weight may improve many of the problems associated with being overweight, such as high blood pressure and diabetes.

How to Reduce Excess Weight

Self-care and wellness depend upon an effective weight management program. This requires that you make a commitment to a healthy diet and an exercise plan. Always remember that understanding the *MindBodySpirit Connection* is the key to successful weight management. As an example, many people overeat and eat the wrong foods in relationship to stress, emotional distress, and memory. As you have learned, this may be located in either the conscious or unconscious *mind.*

Diet

To keep the body weight steady, the amount of calories taken in must be balanced with the amount of calories used by the body. The types and amounts of foods affect ability to maintain weight. High-fat foods have more calories per serving, but people can still gain weight from eating too much of foods that are high in starch, sugars, or protein. Specific dietary recommendations were provided in Chapter 26.

Exercise

All studies now show that you must exercise to be healthy, and that exercise is necessary both to lose weight and to maintain healthy weight. Most Americans spend most of their days and leisure time being inactive. In order to burn calories, less time should be spent on sedentary activities and more time spent on physical activities. Exercise is important to good health and is discussed in the next two chapters (Chapters 29 and 30).

Weight and Fibromyalgia

If you are overweight and have fibromyalgia, then you have an added incentive to commit to a program of balanced diet and exercise. Everyone feels better when he (she) approaches ideal body weight, and reduced weight places less of a strain on the muscles and joints. Your exercise program will not only bring eventual relief from pain and facilitate sleep, but it will also help you to lose the weight and maintain the loss.

Now you are ready to learn about exercise in the next two chapters.

Chapter 29

Exercise

Endurance exercise by itself can be a great stress reducer and source of relaxation. But it has also been my experience that a physical program works best when it's accompanied by a tranquil mind and spirit.

– *It's Better to Believe*
Kenneth Cooper, M.D.
(Father of Aerobics)

For most people, exercise is an essential element of an effective plan for self-care and wellness. Fibromyalgia sufferers have even more to gain from exercise because symptoms can be greatly relieved. However, many who suffer from the illness perceive that their pain and fatigue worsen as they begin exercising. Here is the information you need to overcome this problem and include exercise in your life.

Physical Activity and Public Health

The Centers for Disease Control and Prevention, the American College of Sports Medicine, the National Institutes of Health, and the President's Council on Physical Fitness and Sports have summarized the scientific evidence that links regular physical activity to a variety of physical and mental health benefits (Journal of the American Medical Association. 1995;273:402; and Journal of the American Medical Association 1996; 276:241). Epidemiological research has clearly demonstrated the protective and beneficial effects of physical activity and the risk for several chronic illnesses and diseases, including

- Coronary artery disease
- Hypertension
- Diabetes mellitus
- Osteoporosis
- Osteoarthritis
- Colon cancer
- Breast cancer
- Anxiety
- Depression
- Sleep problems

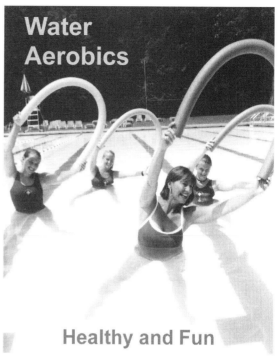

Water Aerobics

Healthy and Fun

Lack of physical activity is correlated with increased all-cause mortality, and it is estimated that 250,000 deaths per year—or 12 percent of all deaths—can be attributed to a lack of regular physical activity.

Finally, weight control that is based upon diet alone without exercise is uniformly unsuccessful (Chapter 28). Exercise is beneficial both in losing and maintaining weight and in converting fat to muscle (Chapter 30).

Physical Activity Recommendations for Adults

- Every U.S. adult should accumulate 30 minutes or more of moderate-intensity physical activity on most, preferably all, days of the week.
- Intermittent activity also confers substantial benefits. The 30 minutes of activity can be accumulated in short bouts of activity, walking up stairs instead of taking the elevator, and walking instead of driving short distances.

Exercise for Osteoarthritis, So Why Not for Fibromyalgia?

Scientific research now shows that exercise is a vital part of the treatment of the "wear and tear" form of osteoarthritis that occurs so commonly with age. The right types of exercise can benefit the joints that have been damaged by osteoarthritis and boost people's overall energy and ability to enjoy the activities of life. Many who have fibromyalgia also have osteoarthritis. Furthermore, if exercise can be so beneficial in the treatment of arthritis, it is reasonable to expect at least the same benefit in fibromyalgia. Read on to see why.

Exercise Can Break the Vicious Cycle

In the past, fibromyalgia was considered to be a muscle disease in which muscle inflammation or impaired blood flow and oxygen delivery to muscles was present. But you now know that fibromyalgia is a *MindBodySpirit Syndrome.* Take a moment to review Chapter 11 on the "cause" of fibromyalgia.

The pain of fibromyalgia results in reduced physical activity and avoidance of exercise. A vicious cycle is established as inactivity and deconditioning lead to increased pain, stiffness, and discomfort and fatigue. Sleep is further impaired, stress management is compromised, and emotional distress is increased. Sleep disturbance, anxiety, and depression amplify and enhance the pain and symptoms of fibromyalgia. Fatigue sets in and exhausts the desire to be active and exercise. The cycle is completed as activity and exercise are further reduced.

Exercise can break this vicious cycle by

- Serving as evidence of the decision to take control
- Improving sleep
- Providing better stress management
- Relieving emotional distress (anxiety and depression)
- Restoring energy
- Relieving pain

Exercise is a natural sleep potion, tranquilizer, antidepressant, and energy tonic!

Exercise and Fibromyalgia: A Unique Challenge

The longest step in the journey is the first, so most people have difficulty motivating themselves to begin a life-long exercise program. It is even more difficult for those who have fibromyalgia because they know from experience that their muscles and joints are more sensitive to pain and that post-exercise discomfort is so discouraging. But they have even more to gain from the journey.

An exercise program will be important in ultimately relieving symptoms as well as in bringing general health benefits. A gradual and incremental exercise program utilizing low impact aerobic activities like fast walking, biking, swimming, or water aerobics are the ones most likely to be initially successful. The type and intensity of the program may need to be individualized, and physical therapists or exercise specialists can provide helpful instruction (Chapter 37).

Physical Trainer

You may choose to work with a qualified physical trainer, at least to begin your program. You may consider your trainer to be a caregiver. Review Chapter 14 on working with a caregiver; you should select a personal trainer as you would a physician. Try to find a trainer who has experience helping people with fibromyalgia.

Important: Get a Medical Examination

It may be important to have your physician's approval before starting an exercise program, depending upon your age and health problems. Without this clearance, an exercise and dietary program could be life threatening if there is an undetected health problem. The NIH consensus panel on exercise has cautioned that people with heart disease, as well as men

187

over age 40 or women over age 50 who have multiple risk factors, should have a medical examination before starting a vigorous exercise program. The examination may not be necessary for those who do not have heart disease or who are not at high risk.

Warm-up and Cooldown

The purpose of the warm-up is to reduce the risk of muscle, ligament, and tendon injury. The exercise should begin with a three-to-five minute warm-up of light calisthenics, walking, cycling, or slow movements which mimic the chosen exercise. For example, if you are walking, your warm-up could be to start the walk at about three-fourths of the speed of your regular workout. Light stretching can also be done. If more demanding stretching is done, it should be done after the warm-up or the cooldown period.

The cooldown is done at the end of the exercise period and should last about five minutes. Walk around slowly, swing your arms, or move otherwise at a slower pace in order to help your body return to a resting state. It is possible to have a serious heart rhythm abnormality if exercise is stopped too suddenly.

The warm-up and cooldown should not count as the 30 or more minutes of exercise.

Two Types of Exercise

Two types of exercise provide different and complementary benefits. The first type of exercise is endurance (aerobic) and will be discussed in this chapter. The second type is resistance (strength) training, which will be discussed in the next chapter. Although both types of exercise are important in a balanced exercise program, we recommend that people with fibromyalgia develop aerobic and endurance fitness first over the course of 3 to 6 months before they move on to resistance (strength) exercise.

Endurance Exercise (Aerobic Exercise)

The term, *aerobics,* was introduced in 1968 by Kenneth Cooper, M.D., in his book *Aerobics.* The book became a quick best seller and sparked the popularity of endurance exercise, leading to the commercial success of celebrities like Jane Fonda and Richard Simmons. Dr. Cooper defines *aerobics* as large-muscle, endurance exercise activity that increases the pulse rate and breathing for a prolonged period of time. The "moderately vigorous exercise" recommended by the NIH and discussed earlier is essentially endurance exercise.

The NIH panel has taken a "middle-of-the-road" approach because it was concerned that the call for more vigorous exercise would discourage the more than 50% of Americans who rarely exercise. However, there is evidence that more strenuous and intense exercise is even more beneficial in reducing the incidence of cardiovascular disease and conferring health benefits. This means that people who already exercise at moderate intensity for at least 30 minutes on most days may benefit from more rigorous exercise like aerobic dancing, step aerobics, stair climbing, fast walking, running, rope skipping, rowing, cycling, and cross-country skiing. Machines like rowers, stationary bicycles, and cross-country ski simulators may also be used.

Just 30 minutes of walking each day has been shown to substantially reduce the risk of disease and can benefit those with fibromyalgia by helping to relieve symptoms. The benefits of walking are cumulative, and three 10-minute walks are equivalent to one 30-minute walk. Of all endurance exercises, walking is the most efficient and effective way to burn fat. It is a weight-bearing activity that exercises the large muscle groups and requires the most calories. Walkers should move fast enough to notice their breathing, but slow enough to be able to carry on a conversation. On average, one hour of brisk walking burns 300 to 450 calories.

How to Tell If Exercise Is Moderately Intense

You can determine whether your exercise is adequate by either measuring your heart rate (pulse), monitoring how you feel, or using a combination of both methods.

Heart rate and pulse

The heart rate is a good indicator of the rate of oxygen consumption and metabolism during exercise, and checking the heart rate is a reasonable way to determine how hard you are exercising. The pulse, or beats per minute, can be taken at the wrist, neck, or by placing the hand over the heart. To get the number of heartbeats per minute, count the number of beats for 15 seconds and multiply that number by 4.

It is not a good idea to get your pulse rate too high while exercising, and an accepted general number for a person's maximum heart rate is 220 minus his (her) age. This number is then used to determine a target heart rate range in order to perform moderately intense exercise.

Moderately intense exercise for both men and women is defined as exercise which maintains the heart rate between 70% and 80% of the maximum heart rate for 30 to 60 minutes.

Example

For a 50-year-old, the heart rate range for moderately intense exercise would be determined as follows:

$$\text{Maximum heart rate} = 220 - \text{age}$$
$$= 220 - 50 = 170 \text{ beats per minute}$$

$$\text{Target heart rate range} = 70\% \text{ to } 80\% \times \text{maximum heart rate}$$
$$= .7(170) \text{ to } .8(170)$$
$$= 119 \text{ to } 136 \text{ beats per minute}$$

So, this 50-year-old person needs to exercise hard enough that the heart beats between 119 and 136 times per minute for 30 to 60 minutes.

A practical approach to determining moderately intense exertion

If you like to avoid math as much as we do, or if you have difficulty measuring the pulse and heart rate during exercise, then you can purchase a heart rate monitor that is worn on the wrist. However, the equation that estimates the maximum heart rate is only accurate for a portion of the population. Thus, there is no perfect way to monitor exercise intensity.

As Dr. Kenneth Cooper says in his book, *It's Better to Believe* (Nashville, TN: Thomas Nelson Inc., 1995), "When you're participating in endurance exercise, you'll experience the greatest fitness benefits if you monitor how you feel about the effort you're putting out. When you first begin, a program should involve at least fairly light effort, and then in later weeks you should move on to a somewhat hard to hard degree of intensity."

So, what does "somewhat hard" to "hard" mean in terms of exertional effort? Consider using what is called the "Borg Rating (Scale) of Perceived Exertion." After gradually increasing exercise and effort for several weeks, most people who exercise and feel that they are working out somewhere in the range of "somewhat hard" to "hard" will meet their goal of endurance exercise benefits. This means that you are aware that you are breathing more rapidly and you may have worked up a sweat but that you could carry on a conversation. Exercising "very hard" feels quite uncomfortable, with a strong sense of fatigue and very labored breathing. It would probably be extremely difficult to carry on a conversation.

Special Instructions for Those with Fibromyalgia

We pointed out that it can be difficult for fibromyalgia sufferers to start and maintain an exercise program; symptoms of pain and fatigue may seem to worsen as they begin their exercise program. By contrast, the value of an exercise program in ultimately bringing symptom relief and conferring general health benefits is substantial. Here are your special instructions.

- **Chart your progress.**   It is worthwhile to record your progress in writing. You will be amazed by how helpful this step can be in maintaining your motivation to continue.

- **Start slowly.**   If you are just beginning your program, you should walk, swim, or cycle for no more than 5 minutes at a time. Do this at least 3 times a day if you can. Your goal will be to exercise on most days for at least 30 minutes.

- **Build gradually.**   Increase the length of your exercise sessions by about 10 percent each week. For example, if you are walking for 10 minutes a day for a week, increase to 11 minutes a day for the next week.

- **Challenge yourself without pushing too hard and becoming discouraged.**   Remember that you are trying to get your heart to pump harder than it does at rest and eventually to break a sweat. You may be somewhat out of breath, but you should be able to carry on a conversation while you exercise.

- **Weight loss is good if overweight.**   Carrying extra body weight is an unnecessary load that can fatigue your muscles and joints faster, so losing even 10% of your body weight can be beneficial. The best strategy for successful and permanent weight loss is exercise, which is combined with healthy eating.

- **Develop endurance fitness before undertaking a resistance (strength) exercise program.**   You will be better prepared to begin building strength and muscle mass.

You are now ready to learn about resistance (strength) exercise in the next chapter.

Chapter 30
Resistance (Strength) Exercise

People don't exercise simply to improve their physical well being
or in an attempt to stay thin or stave off the effects of aging. They
become dedicated to exercise because they find it helps them feel
good emotionally and physically.
— Michael H. Sacks, M.D.
in *Mind Body Medicine* (Goleman and Gurin, Editors)

What is the average woman's number-one fitness problem?
The answer may surprise you. It's the loss of muscle mass.
— *Body Defining*
Ellington Darden, Ph.D.

After developing endurance or aerobic fitness described in the preceding chapter, you will want to move on to building muscle and
strength. Research now shows that you can accomplish the strength
and muscular dimension of your self-care and wellness program in
as little as 20 to 30 minutes, two to three times a week. Strength can
be doubled, fat replaced with muscle—*and most importantly for those
with fibromyalgia—symptoms can be relieved.*

Easy Chair Atrophy: Creeping Obesity and Muscle Loss

Without resistance training, everyone develops what we call "easy chair
atrophy." Most people spend more time with passive entertainment, like
watching sports rather than playing them. They use a golf cart rather than
walk the course and take the car for that short drive rather than walk the

distance. The end result is that most people become fatter and less muscular every year. This is a very unhealthy combination, particularly for those who suffer from fibromyalgia, because it intensifies their symptoms.

Men

Between 20 and 50 years of age, the average man who does not engage in regular strength training exercise loses ½ pound of muscle per year and replaces it with up to 1½ pounds of fat (Figure 30.1). This adds up to 15 pounds of fat gained every ten years and 45 pounds of fat gained in 30 years. This creeping obesity is often disguised by the shrinking muscle mass. Instead of a weight gain of 45 pounds, the loss of 15 pounds of muscle results in only 30 pounds of weight gain. Without resistance exercise training, even if you never gain a pound of weight between your graduation from high school and turning 50 years of age, your body composition will be very different. Fifteen pounds of muscle will have been replaced with 15 pounds of fat. A regular program of resistance training can overcome easy chair atrophy, or creeping obesity.

Fat and Muscle Changes without Exercise

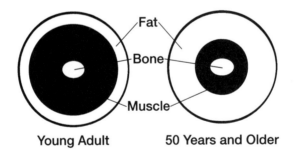

Young Adult   50 Years and Older

Figure 30.1

Women

A woman becomes gradually fatter and less muscular in the same way as the average man does. In 30 years, she gains 30 pounds of weight: 45 pounds are fat, while 15 pounds of muscle are lost (Figure 30.2).

Aging without Exercise: Fatter, Less Muscular

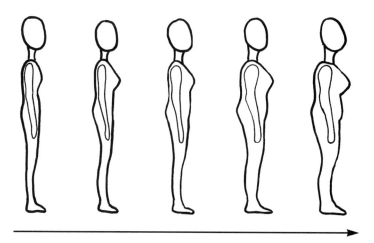

Figure 30.2

The Benefit of Muscle

Muscle is important for both men and women, especially for people who want to lose weight; the muscles of the body burn most of the calories we eat. Each pound of muscle added to the body burns an extra 50 calories per day or 350 calories each week. Adding muscle with strength training increases your *body* metabolism. Muscle is 25 times as active metabolically as is the same amount of fat.

Never Too Late

Scientific studies confirm that resistance training can counteract age-related loss of muscle mass, strength, and general function and convert fat to muscle at any age. Either free weights or machines can be used as long as the large muscle groups are worked beyond levels usually encountered.

The NIH consensus statement recommends that it is important for an exercise program to improve one's ability to perform the activities of life and reduce injury potential. Resistance (strength) training can improve muscular function and can result in some cardiovascular (aerobic) benefits. For the elderly, and those who have been deconditioned from recent inactivity or illness, resistance training can improve their ability to accomplish the tasks of daily living. Resistance training can contribute to better balance, coordination, and agility, which might help prevent falls in the elderly. These abilities also make possible the physical activity that is necessary for aerobic cardiovascular health.

The American College of Sports Medicine recommends strength training two-to-three times a week and flexibility workouts two-to-three times a week.

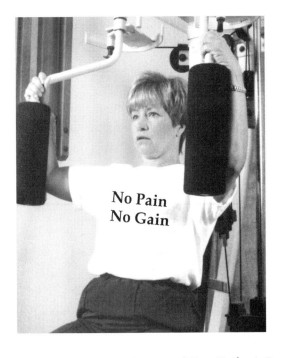

No Pain
No Gain

How to Do Resistance (Strength) Training

Resistance training should be intense in order to actually build and maintain muscle. Arthur Jones, who is the founder of Nautilus® exercise machines, said, "The human body is exercised best, not by the volume of work but rather by the energy put momentarily into that work. Train harder, but briefer."

There are many different books and programs about how to do resistance exercise training. The program that we use and recommend is the one advocated by Ellington Darden, Ph.D., in his books written for men, *Living Longer Stronger* (New York: A Perigee Book, 1995), and for women, *Body Defining* (Chicago: Contemporary Books, 1996). Dr. Darden advocates a very practical strength-training program. According to his exercise regimen, you work all of the major muscle groups on the same day, and you complete the entire workout in 30 minutes or less, two-to-three times a week. You only do one set of each recommended exercise very slowly to the point of momentary muscular failure when the resistance can no longer be moved and another repetition is impossible.

If you are interested in home equipment, Dr. Darden recommends the BOWFLEX machine (1-800-BOWFLEX; www.bowflex.com), which is an exercise system with an adjustable bench attached to a series of vertically positioned power rods. The rods are organized in different levels of resistance and connect to cable-pulley handles. The system can be quickly changed to simulate all of the resistance training exercises.

To Stretch or Not to Stretch?

Although there is some controversy about the benefits of stretching, it is probably a good idea for most people to do some stretching. You can do light stretching as part of your warm-up, but only do more aggressive stretching after the warm-up or during the cool-down period. Research shows that most stretches should be held for at least 30 seconds to provide lasting benefits.

A Final Word on Exercise for Those with Fibromyalgia

If you continue to fear a return of pain after it goes away or if you are worried about activities causing progressive damage to your body, then the pain is likely to return. This is a form of negative programming. You need to overcome these fears in order to heal. Return to normal and unrestricted activity once the pain has gone away and once you believe your diagnosis is correct. This return to activity may take weeks to months, which is perfectly understandable in light of years of misunderstanding about the presumed "weakness" of your body. We recommend that you hold off on your exercise program for at least one month after you finally accept the diagnosis. This permits the pain to diminish, confidence to build, and reprogramming to occur.

Be patient, and begin your exercise program gradually; the resumption of physical activity can be slow and the road bumpy. If exercise brings pain, realize that you cannot hurt yourself and that the process is benign. If pain occurs, consider that it is related to deconditioning and to reprogramming.

You are not only working to eliminate the pain but also to prevent its return in the future. It is the awareness and understanding of the *MindBodySpirit Connection* that brings healing. Be patient and persistent because it can take longer to relieve the fear than the pain.

In the next chapter, you will learn about the effects of alcohol, nicotine, and caffeine on your *mind* and *body.*

Chapter 31
Caffeine, Alcohol, and Nicotine

(Coffee) is the strongest of all the caffeine sources, the
one that is the most irritating to the body, and the one
most associated with addiction.
– *Natural Health, Natural Medicine*
Andrew Weil, M.D.

"On drinking Wine"

1st, Healthy	6th, Revel
2nd, Pleasant	7th, Black eyes
3rd, Soporific	8th, Policemen
4th, Conducive to violence	9th, Biliousness
5th, Uproar	10th, Hurling furniture

– Eubulus (Greco-Roman writer)

A custom loathsome to the eye, hateful to the nose, harmful
to the brain, dangerous to the lungs, and in the black, stinking
fume thereof, nearest resembling the horrible Stygian smoke
of the pit that is bottomless.
– *A Counterblast to Tobacco* (1604)
King James I

Both caffeine and alcohol interfere with REM sleep, which can contribute to the vicious cycle perpetuating the symptoms of fibromyalgia. Furthermore, caffeine is a stimulant which can intensify the pain and fatigue associated with fibromyalgia.

Caffeine

Caffeine is a strong substance found in coffee, tea, chocolate, soft drinks, and in many over-the-counter and prescription medications and drugs. It is a stimulant drug that affects the brain, heart, and GI system. Coca-Cola® syrup containing caffeine was originally developed as a remedy for "sick headache" by a pharmacist. Caffeine potentiates the pain-relieving effects of aspirin or acetaminophen and is added to some prescription headache medications for this reason.

Symptoms and side effects from caffeine

Many people do not realize that caffeine can cause or contribute to the following problems:

- Fibromyalgia
- IBS
- Headache
- Anxiety
- Jittery feelings
- Sleep disturbance
- Fatigue and feeling unwell

The regular use of caffeine can lead to rebound or withdrawal headaches. A 5-ounce cup of coffee typically contains 160 mg of caffeine. Although most Americans consume 200 mg of caffeine each day on average, 15 percent to 20 percent consume more. Some take in over 1000 mg of caffeine per day. Side effects from caffeine usually occur at dosages over 500 mg per day, but they can occur with as little as 250 mg per day.

Caffeine can contribute to anxiety and result in a jittery feeling with actual physical trembling. It can contribute to sleep disturbance, and many people who consult doctors because of problems with rest and sleeping actually have caffeine to blame. This disturbance of sleep can result in fatigue. Therefore, a vicious cycle can develop, as people try to combat fatigue by drinking more coffee. This vicious cycle and aggravation of anxiety contribute to an increased intensity of the symptoms of fibromyalgia.

Table 31.1 lists the most common sources of caffeine. You can see that brewed regular coffee contains the highest amount of caffeine.

Table 31.1

Amounts of Caffeine for Various Sources

Caffeine Sources	Milligrams of Caffeine
Brewed coffee (1 cup)	100–150
Instant coffee (1 cup)	85–100
Decaffeinated coffee (1 cup)	2–4
Tea (1 cup)	30–40
Cocoa (1 cup)	40–55
Cola (8 ounces)	40–60
Chocolate bar	25

Withdrawing from caffeine

Dietary caffeine consumption can be reduced or eliminated by gradually reducing the source of caffeine (coffee or colas, for example). Begin with a 5-ounce reduction of coffee or cola every five to seven days until low doses are reached (100 to 120 mg per day). This dose can be maintained or discontinued altogether. Some people will experience symptoms of caffeine withdrawal from as little as 100 mg per day. Withdrawal from caffeine can take up to a week.

Alcohol

Alcohol can interfere with sleep and aggravate the symptoms of fibromyalgia. Furthermore, excessive alcohol intake can damage muscle and contribute to muscular pain.

Recognition of alcoholism by both patient and doctor can be very difficult because of the delusional denial alcoholics frequently have. Review the screen for alcoholism in Step 4 (Chapter 19). Do you have a problem with alcohol?

Look in the local telephone book Yellow Pages under "Alcoholism Information and Treatment Centers" to find names, addresses, and phone numbers of local 12-step programs (e.g. Alcoholics Anonymous, Alanon) and inpatient and outpatient treatment facilities. Individual programs are also listed in the white pages of the telephone book. For more information about local programs and a catalog of pamphlets and guidelines, contact:

Alcoholics Anonymous World Services, Inc.
PO Box 459
Grand Central Station
New York, New York 10163
(212) 870-3400

The Betty Ford Center
39000 Bob Hope Drive
Rancho Mirage, California 92270
(619) 773-4100 or (800) 854-9211

Nicotine and Tobacco

There is a good reason that all cigarette packs carry the Surgeon General's warning, "Quitting smoking now greatly reduces serious risks to your health." There is probably no habit that is more self-destructive than smoking. Smoking is responsible for several hundred thousand deaths in the United States every year. It is linked to several types of cancer, especially cancer of the lung. It causes and aggravates lung disease including emphysema, chronic bronchitis, and asthma. Finally, smoking is associated with an increased risk of stroke, heart attack, and impaired circulation. Smoking is inconsistent with a plan for self-care and wellness.

How to stop smoking

Studies show that about 70% of smokers have attempted to quit at least once, and that 25% to 50% of current smokers would like to quit. Quitting is difficult, but more than three million Americans are able to do so every year.

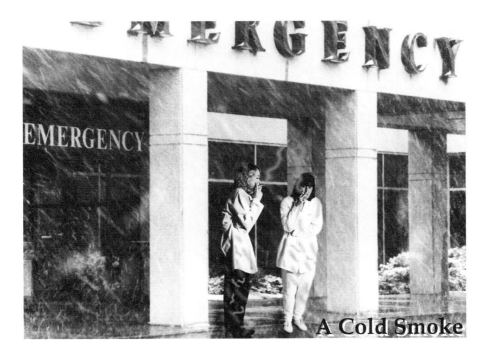

A Cold Smoke

If you want to quit

1. Pick a quitting date sometime within the next two weeks.
2. Use nicotine replacement treatment (either gum or patch) which is available over-the-counter at groceries and pharmacies.
3. Inform family, friends, and coworkers that you are quitting in order to build a support system.

Your doctor can help

Studies clearly show that certain smoking cessation interventions do work and that doctors can help smokers to overcome the physical addiction to nicotine and psychological addiction to tobacco (see first listing in "Resources" at the end of the chapter).

Bupropion is an atypical antidepressant called Wellbutrin® (Chapter 23). It has recently been approved for assistance to smokers in quitting the habit and is called Zyban®.

After you have stopped

Consider talking to your doctor within the first week or two to receive positive reinforcement and encouragement. Discuss any withdrawal symptoms, cravings, irritability, and weight gain, and schedule another visit with the doctor for one month and later, if needed.

Problems along the way

Drinking alcohol or living or working with others who smoke can derail attempts to quit smoking. Make some changes (such as asking others who smoke not to smoke in your presence) in order to reduce your risk of failure. Don't be too discouraged if a relapse occurs; try again. Consider an intense smoking-cessation program, which can be a more effective way to achieve the long-term goal of nicotine abstinence.

Be aware that it is common for people to gain weight after quitting smoking. Use this opportunity to begin your exercise program. Some dietary changes might also be necessary, such as avoiding the temptation to snack instead of smoking a cigarette. Long-term studies show that men gain an average of 6 pounds after they quit smoking, and women gain an average of 8 pounds. About 10% of men and 15% of women gain nearly 30 pounds.

If you don't want to quit

Look again at all of the risks of smoking, and look at your own medical situation as it relates to smoking. Review the benefits of quitting: better self-care, wellness and health, freedom from addiction, and better tasting food. Finally, both you and your surroundings will no longer smell of smoke.

Resources

Agency for Health Care Policy and Research (AHCPR)   The American Medical Association (AMA) and the Agency for Health Care Policy and Research (AHCPR)—an agency of the federal government—have developed a program entitled *Smoking Cessation Guide for Primary Care Clini-*

cians. It is a systematic, practical, and evidence-based approach to stopping tobacco use. In case your doctor does not have the program, it is available free of charge from the AHCPR Publications Clearinghouse:

Smoking Cessation
PO Box 8547
Silver Spring, MD 20907-8547
Telephone (800) 358-9295

The program can be immediately obtained by:

AHCPR Instant Fax (301) 594-2800
AHCPR http://www.ahcpr.gov/clinic under Clinical Practice
   Guidelines

The National Institutes of Health (National Cancer Institute) publishes a pamphlet, "Clearing the Air: How to Quit Smoking . . . and Quit for Keeps," NIH Publication No. 95-1647, revised September 1993, reprinted September 1995. Call the Cancer Information Service, a program of the National Cancer Institute at 1-800-4-Cancer (1-800-422-6237).

American Cancer Society (ACS) is a voluntary organization that assists people in learning about the health hazards of smoking and becoming successful ex-smokers. They hold a "Great American Smokeout" in November and the Annual Cancer Crusade in April, and publish numerous educational materials. American Cancer Society, 1599 Clifton Road, NE, Atlanta, GA 30329, (404) 320-3333.

American Heart Association (AHA) is a voluntary organization that produces many publications and audiovisual materials about the harmful effects of smoking on the heart. The AHA also has a guidebook for incorporating a weight-control component into smoking cessation programs. American Heart Association, 7272 Greenville Avenue, Dallas, TX 75231, (214) 373-6300.

American Lung Association (ALA) is a voluntary organization that provides help for smokers who want to quit through their Freedom from Smoking Self-help Smoking Cessation Program. The organization actively supports legislation and information campaigns for nonsmokers' rights and conducts public information programs about the health effects of smoking. American Lung Association, 1740 Broadway, New York, NY 10019-4374, (212) 315-8700.

Office on Smoking and Health (OSH) is the Department of Health and Human Services lead agency in smoking control. OSH sponsors distribution of publications on smoking-related topics, such as free flyers on relapse after initial quitting, helping a friend or family member quit smoking, the health hazards of smoking, and the effects of parental smoking on teenagers. Office on Smoking and Health, Centers for Disease Control, Mail Stop K-50, 4770 Buford Highway, NE, Atlanta, GA 30341-3724, (404) 488-5705.

Take the next step to learn more about what you can do about your illness.

REVIEW OF STEP 5

1. Health and wellness are your responsibility; do not assume you will remain healthy. Self-care is an active, not a passive process.

2. Sleep is important in relief from symptoms and in maintaining wellness.

3. Expert opinion remains divided about whether taking antioxidant vitamins in dosages higher than the recommended RDA confers additional benefits.

4. Know how these six main nutritional issues can affect you: fat-cholesterol, carbohydrate, fiber, protein, calcium, and supplements (including vitamins, antioxidants, and minerals).

5. Obesity is the second leading cause of preventable death in the U.S. (after smoking). If you have a high Body Mass Index (BMI), take steps to reduce your weight through healthy diet and exercise.

6. Incorporate moderate exercise into your daily routine. Include both endurance (aerobic) and resistance (strength) exercise. Exercise can be beneficial even if it is done in ten-minute spurts.

7. Restricting alcohol use to moderation (if you drink at all) and not smoking are two factors you can control to improve your overall health. Caffeine restriction can be beneficial, particularly if anxiety is present. Use the resources listed for help if this is a problem for you.

STEP 6

MANAGING YOUR FIBROMYALGIA

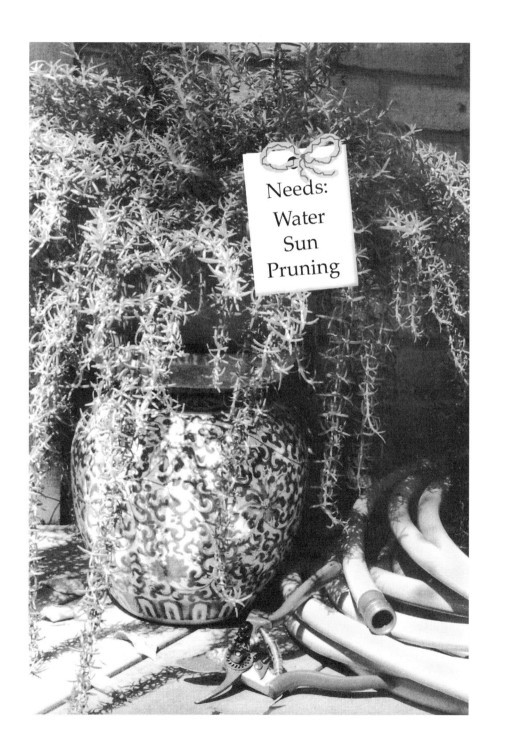

Needs:
Water
Sun
Pruning

Chapter 32

Trigger (Tender) Point Injections; Spray and Stretch

> The physician is only nature's assistant.
> – Galen

Local therapy directed to painful areas may be helpful in the treatment of fibromyalgia.

Trigger (Tender) Point Injections

There have been very few scientific studies of trigger or tender point injections in the treatment of fibromyalgia. Injections are actually used more often in the treatment of localized myofascial pain syndrome (Chapter 10). Although such treatment is somewhat controversial, many doctors find the technique to be useful in relieving the localized pain of fibromyalgia (myofascial pain).

These injections are primarily used in the back, neck, and to a lesser degree, the arms and legs. The doctor palpates—or feels for—tender points within the muscle. The tender point is often no larger than the tip of the doctor's finger. Once the tender point is identified, the doctor uses a syringe filled with either (1) an anesthetic (a numbing drug), (2) a combination of an anesthetic and a corticosteroid, or (3) saline (salt water) alone. The injection is made into the tender point with a needle attached to the syringe.

It is somewhat amazing that the content of the syringe does not seem to matter in terms of beneficial results. What seems to be most important is how close to the tender point the injection is. The doctor tries to aim for the point of maximum tenderness. Some doctors actually use a "dry needle" without injecting anything and get the same benefits.

The injection may be uncomfortable for a moment, but then numbness sets in when an anesthetic is used. Pain is relieved and then the muscle can be stretched and massaged. This is called myofascial release. Pain relief can last for weeks to months, and injections can be repeated. However, corticosteroids can have harmful effects when repeatedly used.

Spray and Stretch Therapy

This technique can be performed independently or along with trigger point injections. A vapocoolant spray, usually fluorimethane or ethyl chloride, is applied to the skin over the tender point. The muscle is then passively stretched. Initially, there may be some pain and discomfort. As the process continues, pain decreases, trigger point tenderness is reduced, and range of motion of the nearby joint may increase if it had been restricted.

Medications are described in the next chapter.

Chapter 33
Medications

It's really a very simple idea: no prescription
is worth more than knowledge.
– C. Everett Koop, M.D.
(Former Surgeon General of the United States)

Fibromyalgia is a *MindBodySpirit Syndrome*. If medications are necessary, this chapter will help you to understand how they can help.

Anti-inflammatory and Analgesic Medications

You now know that the muscles and tissues are not inflamed in fibromyalgia, so it should not be much of a surprise that anti-inflammatory medications are not very effective in treatment. Nonsteroidal anti-inflammatory drugs (NSAIDs) like ibuprofen and naproxen, as well as more powerful anti-inflammatory medication called corticosteroid (e.g., prednisone), have not been shown to be any more effective than a placebo in scientific studies. But, NSAIDs may have an additive effect when they are combined with central nervous system (CNS) active medications (see below), and they do have some analgesic effect independent of anti-inflammatory action. Acetaminophen may be helpful, but prolonged use of narcotic analgesics should be avoided because of potential addiction.

Central Nervous System (CNS) Active Medications

Medications that are active in the CNS (brain) include antidepressants (Chapter 23) and cyclobenzaprine (Flexeril®). These drugs have been shown to be of some value in scientific studies. Cyclobenzaprine and Carisoprodol (Soma®) are considered to be muscle relaxants, but it is likely that any benefit derives mainly from their CNS effects.

Furthermore, various combinations of CNS active medications may be more useful than any single drug. For example, one study found that the combination of 20 mg of fluoxetine (Prozac®) in the morning with 25 mg of amitriptyline (Elavil®) at bedtime was more effective than either medication used alone.

Tramadol (Ultram®) is a drug that binds to opiate receptors in the brain, which inhibits the transmission of pain signals to the brain through ascending pathways. This alters the perception of and response to pain. The ascending pain pathway is further modified by alteration of serotonin and norepinephrine reuptake (Chapters 4 and 23).

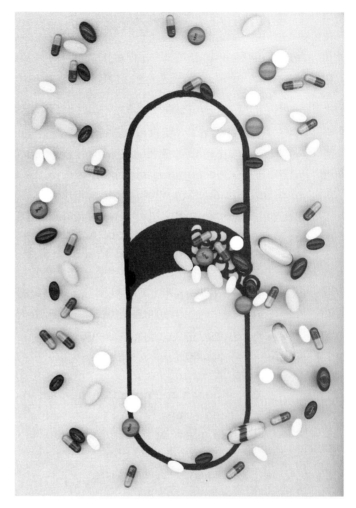

Patients with associated nighttime myoclonus or repetitive limb movements may be helped by low doses of benzodiazepines, such as clonazepam, 0.5 mg at bedtime (Chapter 25).

Guaifenesin (glyceryl guaicolate)

Guaifenesin is a safe ingredient found in many cough and cold remedies. R. Paul St. Amand, M.D., recommends guaifenesin as a treatment for fibromyalgia, based upon his theories and experience (*What Your Doctor May Not Tell You about Fibromyalgia*, New York: Warner Books, 1999). His regimen requires strict avoidance of salicylates, which are found in many substances that range from cosmetics (including lipsticks), sunscreens, deodorants, and aspirins to herbs and plant juices (absorbed through the skin while gardening).

Although many fibromyalgia patients have been helped by Dr. St. Amand and his treatment plan, a recent scientific study conducted by Robert M. Bennett, M.D., Professor of Medicine and Chairman of the Division of Arthritis and Rheumatic Diseases, Oregon Health Sciences University, Portland, Oregon, has provided persuasive evidence that guaifenesin has no beneficial action by itself in the treatment of fibromyalgia (http://www. myalgia.com).

We agree with Dr. Bennett's comments that the real benefits reported by Dr. St. Amand are most likely explained by a placebo response, where guaifenesin is a potent focus in a program of cognitive behavioral therapy. Dr. Amand's empathy, enthusiasm, and charisma play an important role as well. In our view, his results are further evidence of the remarkable healing power found within the biopsychosocialspiritual approach and the *MindBodySpirit Connection*.

Summary

If medication is needed, we usually start patients on a low dose of a tricyclic antidepressant medication at bedtime and use simple analgesics as needed during the day. If response is inadequate, another antidepressant drug may either be added or substituted. When these medications begin to take effect, the symptoms of pain, fatigue, and altered sleep improve. Then, stretching and exercise can be initiated. Of course, everyone is different, and it is necessary to individualize treatment over time.

Chapter 34

Support Groups

Meeting other patients with fibromyalgia syndrome, particularly
in the context of an educational seminar, is often a benefit in
gaining a greater self-understanding.
– Robert Bennett, M.D.

Most people with fibromyalgia want to learn as much about their
condition as possible in order to better cope and recover. Support
groups and networks composed of other fibromyalgia patients can
be a valuable educational and motivational resource.

Advantages of belonging to a support group include

- Facilitating healing (review Chapter 12)
- Receiving emotional and moral support
- It is helpful to know that you are not alone and that there are many
  others who struggle with the same problem that you have. You can
  see how other people manage their problems and learn from them.
  This mutual support can be the key to your recognition of your own
  power and responsibility.
- Learning about the latest scientific information
- Taking advantage of opportunities to read and hear from physicians
  and other health care professionals and have questions answered
- Identifying local support groups or chapters, doctors, and other
  health professionals in your community

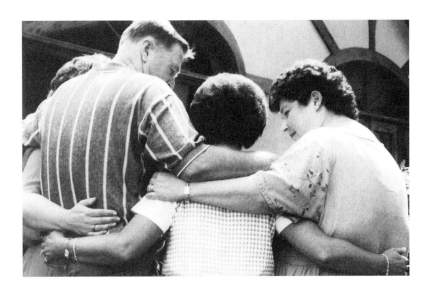

Here is a listing of support groups.

Arthritis Foundation
1330 W. Peachtree St.
Atlanta, GA 30309
(404) 872-7100
www.arthritis.org

The Fibromyalgia Alliance of America, Inc.
PO Box 21990
Columbus, OH 43221-0990
(888) 717-6711
(614) 457-4222
Fax (614) 457-2729
Contact Mary Anne Saathoff, RN
(No Web site located)

Fibromyalgia Association-USA
PO Box 20408
Columbus, OH 43220
www.fibromyalgiaassnusa.org

American Fibromyalgia Syndrome Association, Inc. (AFSA)
6380 Tanque Verde
Suite D
Tucson, AZ 85715
(520) 733-1570
www.afsafund.org

National Fibromyalgia Research Organization
PO Box 500
Salem, OR 97302
www.teleport.com/~nfra/

National Institute of Arthritis and Musculoskeletal
   and Skin Diseases (NIAMS)
1 AMS Circle
Bethesda, MD 20892-3675
(301) 495-4484
Fax (301) 587-4352
www.nih.gov/niams/healthinfo/fibromya.htm

Fibromyalgia Network
PO Box 31750
Tucson, AZ 85751-1750
(800) 853-2929
(520) 290-5508
Fax (520) 290-5550
http://fmnetnews.com
Contact: Ms. Kristin Thorson

We will "sum it all up" in the next chapter.

Chapter 35

Summing It All Up

We have met the enemy and he is us.
– Pogo
Walt Kelly

> It is not simply *mind* over matter *(body)*, but clearly mind does matter.

That Was Then

The pain developed so gradually that you cannot recall how and when it began. It might have started with an accident, injury, or infection. You might have found that the pain was worse during either the day or the night. It might have been more severe when you first got out of bed and better as the day wore on. By contrast, the pain might have become progressively more severe throughout the day. Pain might have been either improved or aggravated by standing, walking, or sitting. In addition, the pain might have occurred at totally unpredictable times and not have occurred when you expected it to.

You might have feared certain activities and positions and been afraid to lift anything or bend over. Your pain, avoidance of activities, and fear might have interfered with your ability to do your job or work at home. You might have decided not to exercise or play in sports because of the pain and fear. Or if you still played, you did so in spite of the pain.

You have been fatigued and have trouble sleeping. Usually, sleep would not relieve the weariness.

You could not understand how you could have so many different symptoms that have been diagnosed by several different doctors as syndromes, such as tension headache syndrome, irritable bowel syndrome, chronic pelvic pain syndrome, and irritable bladder syndrome. You have not been able to obtain relief either.

You might or might not be aware of a relationship between stress, emotional distress (anxiety or depression), or painful memories and your pain.

This Is Now

Now you know that even though your fibromyalgia might have been triggered by an injury, accident, or infection, the damage is not permanent. You know that you do not have a chronic infection or inflammation condition causing your symptoms. Now that you are diagnosed with fibromyalgia, you understand that you have many tender areas—called trigger points—that are expected in fibromyalgia.

You understand that you do not have another disease or disorder that could be mimicking fibromyalgia. Your tests are probably normal. However, if any structural findings are found on your tests, such as arthritis on an x-ray, you are reassured that they are commonly found in most of us as we age and that they are not the cause of your pain. If you do have both fibromyalgia and another condition such as arthritis, you understand that treatment of fibromyalgia is as important or more so than the treatment of the coexisting condition.

You know that you are so uncomfortable with the pain that you have reduced your activity and have not felt that you could exercise. All of this has resulted in physical deconditioning and poor fitness. You know that a vicious cycle has become established as inactivity and deconditioning lead to increased pain, stiffness, and discomfort and further disturbance of sleep, mood, and energy.

You know that the pain of fibromyalgia is real and not imagined. It can be intense, but it is harmless and will not damage your body—now or when it finally goes away. Even though it is not "all in your head," the head contains an organ, the *mind* (brain), which is playing an important role in the cause through the *MindBodySpirit Connection.* The tension in your muscles is not coming from inflammation or a disease process. There is an abnormality of pain perception and reception at the *mind* (brain) level and perhaps an increased sensitivity of the muscles themselves.

You realize that your fatigue and difficulty sleeping are also *MindBody-Spirit Symptoms.* You know that fibromyalgia and any other functional syndromes that you are diagnosed with, like chronic headache, irritable bowel syndrome, chronic pelvic pain, or an irritable bladder, are *Mind-BodySpirit Syndromes.*

Now you appreciate how essential it is to recognize, accept, and address the management of stress, emotional distress, and memory. Now you see how conscious stress, emotion (like anxiety and depression), and painful memories (for example, having been abused), can intensify symptoms and reduce coping ability. You realize that unconscious stress, emotional distress, and memories may even be at the root of the problem. You are beginning to understand that it is the acceptance of this and not necessarily the identification of the stress, emotional distress, or memory that can be therapeutic.

Focus upon Healing

Review and renew your commitment to *MindBodySpirit Healing.*

- Review the biopsychosocialspiritual model of illness, disease, and wellness.
- Remember that there is a difference between illness and disease and between treatment and healing.
- Know that understanding the *MindBodySpirit Connection* is therapeutic.
- Realize that it is normal to have *MindBodySpirit Symptoms.* Everyone has them and it is not an indication of weakness or mental illness.

- Appreciate that fibromyalgia is a collection of *MindBodySpirit Symptoms* that we call a *MindBodySpirit Syndrome.* There are many other similar syndromes that commonly occur with fibromyalgia, such as irritable bowel syndrome.

- De-emphasize any findings that may be found on tests; fibromyalgia is most likely unrelated to them. Do not allow the nocebo effect to affect you and interfere with your healing.

- Accept that conscious and unconscious stress, emotional distress, thoughts, and memory are playing a role in your illness. Stress management, treatment of anxiety and depression, changing the way you think about things, and true acceptance of all this will be therapeutic and bring healing.

- Be optimistic that sleep disturbance can be lessened or eliminated and that this will help to relieve symptoms.

- Commit to an exercise plan in order to break the vicious cycle that has become established as a result of inactivity and deconditioning. This has led to increased pain, stiffness, and discomfort and further disturbance of sleep, mood, and energy. You will break the cycle through conditioning, improved sleep and mood, and increased energy. Exercise is a natural sleep potion, tranquilizer, and anti-depressant!

- Take medication if you need it, and accept that antidepressants can be used as pain relievers, even if depression is not present. If you are depressed or anxious, accept treatment without guilt and be optimistic. You will most likely be able to stop taking medications as you heal.

And if you are still not on the road to recovery and healing, take the next step.

REVIEW OF STEP 6

1. Your doctor may be able to help you by injecting trigger (tender) points with medication.

2. Spray and stretch techniques may bring some relief from pain.

3. Some medications may be helpful. Remember that antidepressant drugs can be used for pain and symptom relief.

4. Consider joining a fibromyalgia support group.

5. Review Chapter 35, "Summing It All Up."

STEP 7

TAKING ACTION IF SYMPTOMS PERSIST

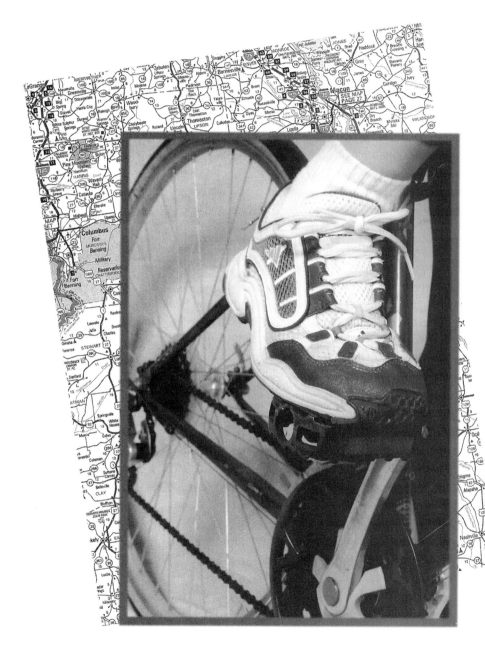

Chapter 36

Specialists

The greatest mistake in the treatment of disease is that there
are physicians for the body and physicians for the soul, although
the two cannot be separated.

– Plato

Most likely, you have been seeing a primary care physician, either a
family practice or internal medicine doctor. This is the best place to
start. But specialists may be helpful, particularly if you are not making progress.

How Healing Occurs

Not all physicians have a good understanding of how to advise patients
with fibromyalgia and other *MindBodySpirit Symptoms* and *MindBody-
Spirit Syndromes.* You should be able to tell if your doctor is interested
in you and is trying to help you. Refer to Step 3, "Healing with Diagnosis and Education." If you are not able to develop a partnership and
treatment plan which relieves your symptoms, you might want to ask
for a referral or consult with a specialist or a Center of Excellence (see
Chapter 41).

Physician Specialists

The following are the physician specialists that may offer special expertise
in fibromyalgia.

Neurologist

A neurologist is an expert in conditions involving the brain, spinal cord, and peripheral nerves. Patients often see neurologists in order to be certain that they do not have a neurologic disorder either mimicking or co-existing with fibromyalgia (see Chapter 15).

Orthopedic surgeon

An orthopedic surgeon is a surgeon and expert in both surgical and nonsurgical management of injuries, diseases, and illnesses involving the neck, back, arms, and legs. Many people think of orthopedic surgeons relative to sports and recreational injuries. Orthopedic surgeons are skilled in the recognition and differential diagnosis of fibromyalgia but may differ in interest in working with patients ultimately diagnosed with fibromyalgia. They may refer the patient with fibromyalgia to other specialists.

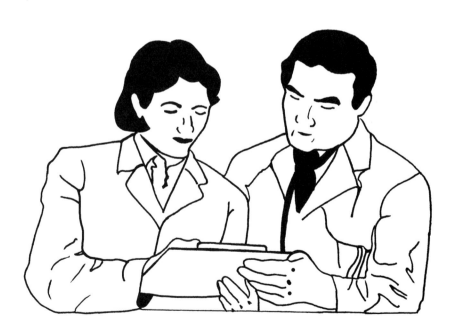

Pain management specialists (anesthesiologists)

These specialists evaluate and treat patients with acute and chronic pain of many different diseases and causes. The pain management specialist orders treatment that may include medication, physical therapy, nerve blocks, psychological counseling, and even surgery.

Physiatrists (physical medicine and rehabilitation specialists)

These doctors are experts in the nonsurgical management of musculo-skeletal conditions and rehabilitation of disabling conditions. Most physical medicine specialists are interested in fibromyalgia and work closely with their patients. They also are skilled in the use of certain types of specialized diagnostic tests, such as electromyography and nerve conduction studies to evaluate nerve and muscle function. They work closely with physical and occupational therapists.

Rheumatologist

Rheumatologists are internal medicine subspecialists who diagnose and treat patients with arthritis, connective tissue disorders, and fibromyalgia.

Other medical professionals are discussed in the next chapter.

Chapter 37

Other Professionals and Caregivers

Indeed, no leap is possible: not because of an unbridgeable
gulf between mind and body, but because at the archaic level
the body is the mind.
— *Love and Its Place in Nature: A Philosophical
Interpretation of Freudian Psychoanalysis*
Jonathan Lear (philosopher-analyst)

Caregivers other than physicians may be able to help in the management of fibromyalgia.

Physical Therapists

Physical therapists are usually very knowledgeable about fibromyalgia. They can help patients find the best combination of therapy and exercise.

Physical therapy can include application of cold or heat to painful areas of the body, massage, ultrasound stimulation, whirlpool therapy, electrical stimulation, stretching and range of motion exercise, and exercise instruction. Exercise is discussed in Chapters 29 and 30.

We feel that physical therapy may be useful, although not essential, for some patients with fibromyalgia in order to reduce pain and while they work through the initial phases of treatment. Once exercise and therapy results in overall improvement in conditioning and general health, this knowledge can then be transferred to a self-directed, home-based program that becomes part of an overall self-care and wellness agenda.

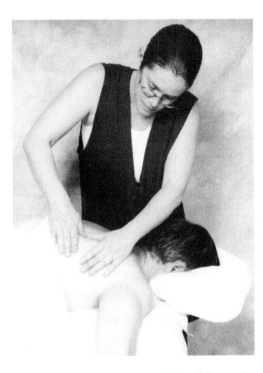

Manual Therapists

The term, "manual therapy" translates literally to treatment with the hands. For centuries, healing has been associated with the use of the hands. There are many references and stories of healing by a practitioner through the "laying on of hands." Some feel that conventional modern medicine as applied by physicians (referred to as allopathic medicine) has lost "touch" with patients by failing to include manipulation and massage in treatment programs for fibromyalgia. Practitioners that include manipulation and massage include chiropractors, massage therapists, osteopaths (DOs), physical therapists, and others.

The goal of all of these therapists should be the same: to provide pain relief and improvement in flexibility of muscles and joints. Manipulation and massage usually bring some relief for a while, and meditation (Chapter 21) can be practiced during massage. However, they are not a substitute for a holistic self-care plan that includes exercise and better sleep. If you decide to work with a manual therapist, it is important that you work with one who has an appropriate professional education and experience with fibromyalgia. Review Chapters 12, 13, and 14 regarding the healing process and the importance of your relationship with the professional.

If you still have not made satisfactory progress, the next chapter will guide you in revisiting relevant sections of the book.

Chapter 38

Stress, Emotional Distress, Thoughts, and Memory

The greatest revolution of our time is the knowledge that human beings, by changing the inner attitudes of their minds, can transform the outer aspects of their lives.
– William James

It may be necessary for you to revisit the impact of stress, emotional distress, and memory in the *MindBodySpirit Connection.*

Be Honest with Yourself

We recommend that you review Step 1 and take the self-tests in Chapter 19. If you have not done so, keep a journal as described in Chapter 20. Review stress management in Chapter 21.

Cognitive Behavioral Therapy

The healthy approach to the management of chronic pain and symptoms requires the exploration of the connection and relationship of thoughts and feelings. The mind gives meaning to experience, including symptoms and pain. Therefore, a despondent, hopeless, self-defeated thinking contributes to negative interpretation of symptoms and pain signals, which increases discomfort, distress, and despair. Remember that the mind is a "filter" or "lens" through which the symptom and pain message and signal transmission pass. The filter or lens can either reduce or magnify the intensity of the message.

Review cognitive techniques described in Chapter 22, which can allow you to explore what determines how you see the world around you and interpret what happens to you. Cognitive behavioral therapy is oriented to correcting thinking and thoughts that are "automatic" and counterproductive. These techniques can be learned, either by working with a health-care professional or by using materials, such as Dr. Margaret Caudill's book, *Managing Pain Before It Manages You* (New York: The Guilford Press, 1995). Another recent book that we can recommend is *Life Strategies: Doing What Works; Doing What Matters,* by Phillip C. McGraw, Ph.D. (New York: Hyperion, 1999).

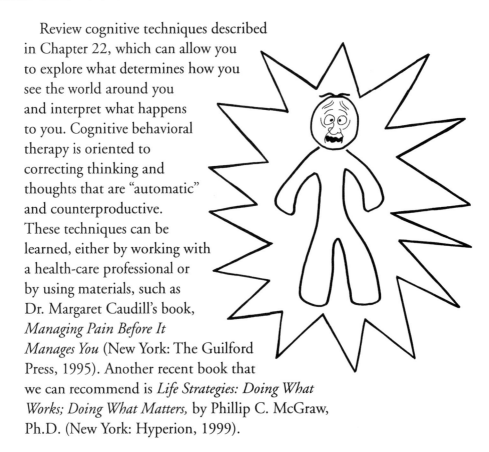

Medication

Remember that antidepressant drugs can be very helpful in chronic pain conditions (Chapter 23). They can act as pain relievers operating at the brain level, even in doses lower than are necessary to treat depression. If there is associated depression, then full antidepressant doses are used; low doses used to treat chronic pain are usually not sufficient to treat depression.

If you want to explore alternative and complementary therapies, then read the next two chapters.

Chapter 39

Alternative and Complementary Medicine

Mind/body medicine is not so much an "alternative" approach as a complementary one. It is perfectly compatible with standard medicine and can be a powerful way of augmenting it, not challenging it or replacing it.

— *Mind Body Medicine*
Dan Goleman, Ph.D., and Joel Gurin, Editors

More and more people are turning to treatments of illness and disease that are not based on traditional Western methods.

Definitions

Alternative medicine refers to remedies and techniques that are unproved. Alternative therapies are an international phenomenon, flourishing in United States, Asia, Australia, Europe, and Canada. They are called *complementary therapies* in many countries because they are used in addition to conventional treatments. Alternative and complementary therapy systems (homeopathy, osteopathy, chiropractic, and Western herbalism), approaches (healing touch, aromatherapy, and light therapy), and integrated and traditional systems (naturopathic medicine, Chinese medicine, Ayurveda, and curanderismo) are widespread.

Interest in the United States

In 1997, 83 million Americans—more than 40% of the adult population—consulted with herbalists, chiropractors, and other unconventional practitioners. More visits to these healers (629 million) were made than to primary care physicians (386 million). The total cost was a whopping $27 billion. By comparing this survey result with one published in the New England Journal of Medicine in 1993, Harvard's Dr. David Eisenberg has confirmed that the interest in alternative and complementary therapy has escalated markedly. Reliance on alternative practitioners—including homeopaths, hypnotists, and herbalists—has grown by nearly 50% during the 1990s.

In November of 1998, the American Medical Association devoted all 10 of its journals, including the centerpiece, *Journal of the American Medical Association,* to articles on alternative treatments.

What Options Are Available?

Alternative medicine has been recognized by mainstream medicine. An Office of Alternative Medicine (OAM) was established at the National Institutes of Health in 1992 by congressional mandate. It has been renamed as the National Center for Complementary and Alternative Medicine. The subject of alternative and complementary medicine is a large one with considerable controversy and mystery. The Center groups the alternative therapies into seven categories:

1. Diet and nutrition
2. Mind-body techniques
3. Bioelectromagnetics
4. Alternative systems of medical practice (or traditional and folk remedies)
5. Pharmacologic and biologic treatments
6. Manual healing methods
7. Herbal medicine

As an example, category 4 is based upon ancient systems of healing which are in turn based upon concepts of human physiology different from those accepted by modern Western science. Two of the most popular healing systems are traditional Chinese medicine with its focus on chi, the life force, and India's Ayurveda ("life knowledge"), popularized by best-selling author Deepak Chopra, M.D.

In March, 1996, The Food and Drug Administration declared that acupuncture needle therapy can be useful, although it did not endorse its use in the treatment of specific disorders. Since then, it has been approved for certain applications, including chronic pain. Research on acupuncture is proceeding at many medical centers in the United States, and evidence is accumulating that the ancient healing art can be helpful.

Integrated Medicine

The economic forces of managed care and the worldwide consumer demand for natural and alternative therapies are not to be denied. Harvard-trained Andrew Weil, M.D., calls for *integrated medicine.* This is a blend of the best of both worlds by promoting health and healing through the integration of the best concepts and techniques of both allopathic and alternative/complementary medicine. It neither rejects conventional medicine nor embraces alternative medicine uncritically. There will be an increasing emphasis by everyone, including doctors and insurance companies, upon comprehensive lifestyle changes.

The next chapter discusses specific natural treatments that have become popular.

Chapter 40

Specific Natural Treatments

I hope that you no longer feel (if indeed you ever did) that
accepting the reality of mental influences on health means
suspending your disbelief and signing up to some dubious
brand of alternative medicine.
– *The Healing Mind*
Paul Martin, Ph.D.

In such a night
Medea gathered the enchanted herbs
that did renew old Aeson.
– *The Merchant of Venice*
Shakespeare

Unfortunately, conventional medicine has not been successful
enough in the treatment of fibromyalgia to satisfy the public. At
least some of the benefits of alternative medicine can be attributed
to the placebo effect, but the placebo effect tends to be temporary
and not curative. Furthermore, the alternative treatment places the
focus upon the *body* rather than the *MindBodySpirit Connection.*

If You Go There

Seek out those who, like Andrew Weil, M.D., teach that each of us has
a capacity for self-healing and that we are, as Norman Cousins said,
"stronger than we think." Place the emphasis upon the *MindBodySpirit
Connection* and consider herbals as only one element of a comprehensive
lifestyle change as illustrated in this book. Form a strong relationship with

your physician or healer, understand the placebo and nocebo effects, commit to a healthy diet and exercise program, and achieve and maintain a healthy body weight. Have a program of stress management, accept the impact of stress, emotion, and memory upon your body, try cognitive behavioral therapy, take traditional medications if you need them, and consider integrating religion/spirituality into your life.

If you take an herb or an alternative treatment, know that you may only realize a temporary placebo effect at best. Scientific evaluation of the efficacy of alternative treatments is underway, so it should become easier to remain up to date and select those therapies that might be of value.

The Food and Drug Administration does not check herbal remedies for quality, safety, and efficacy, and most have not been formally tested for side effects. You will begin to see that the better brands conform to standards of content and purity. Major pharmaceutical companies are just beginning to market herbal preparations.

If you are using alternative or complementary treatments, be sure to let your doctor know about it. Studies show that most people do not do this. Medication prescribed by your doctor could conflict with an alternative or complementary therapy.

We include the most commonly used alternative therapies that may be helpful in the treatment of fibromyalgia.

Specific Therapies

Boswellia: *for muscular pain*

This is an Ayurvedic medicine that is touted for treatment of generalized inflammatory conditions. Although it is advocated for treatment of the pain of fibromyalgia, remember that there is no inflammation present in the condition.

Ginger: *for muscular pain*

Ginger is a spice that is often recommended for treatment of musculoskeletal pain. It is available as tea, ginger root, candied ginger, or as a honey-based syrup. Powdered extracts in capsules and alcohol extracts of ginger are also available.

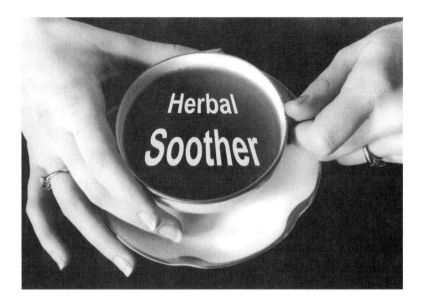

Kava: for anxiety and muscular relaxation

Kava is the root of a tropical shrub in the black-pepper family. It is supposed to relax muscles without loss of mental clarity.

S-adenosyl-methionine (SAMe): for arthritis and depression

S-adenosyl-methionine is also known as SAMe and has been sold in Europe for over 20 years as a prescription treatment for arthritis and depression. It is now available in the United States as an over-the-counter dietary supplement. SAMe is not an herb; rather, it is a chemical that our bodies manufacture from methionine, an amino acid found in foods rich in protein.

St. John's wort: for depression

St. John's wort, or hypericum perforatum, is a very popular herbal treatment in Europe for mild to moderate depression. It has received much attention in the United States. At this writing, the National Institutes of Health is involved in a large multicenter clinical trial to determine whether St. John's wort is truly helpful in treatment of depression.

St. John's wort is available over-the-counter at a recommended dosage of 300 mg, containing 0.3% hypericin, three times a day. It may take as long as six weeks to take effect and seems to be remarkably safe.

Turmeric: for muscular pain

Turmeric is a yellow spice that colors curry and American mustard. An extract of turmeric called curcumin is available in health food stores.

Valerian: for sleeping aid, calming agent

Valerian was the main sedative used in Europe and America before the invention of barbiturate drugs in the early part of this century. The root of the plant has a distinctive odor that some people find to be disagreeable. Valerian is milder than sleeping medications prescribed by doctors but probably should not be used along with prescription hypnotic drugs.

5-HTP (5-hydroxytryptophan): for depression and sleep problems

This is a natural compound that is produced by the body from tryptophan, an amino acid found in many foods. 5-HTP is a precursor of a neurotransmitter called serotonin (Chapter 4). 5-HTP has been used for many years in Europe as a treatment for depression and sleep problems.

Chronic pain management and "Centers of Excellence" are discussed in the next chapter.

Chapter 41

Chronic Pain Management and Centers of Excellence

> Don't deny the diagnosis. Try to deny the verdict.
> – *Head First, The Biology of Hope*
> Norman Cousins

> People who have chronic pain of any type may only be able to "see"
> the world by what the *mind* "allows" them to experience.

The Strain of Pain

The effort to cope with the pain leads to stress-related symptoms, fatigue, sleep difficulties, and problems with appetite and weight control. Relationships with other people can suffer. Fear, anxiety, increased physical tension, and depression are common and can actually increase the pain. A vicious circle perpetuates the problem: pain as chronic stress leads to psychological problems, which leads to more pain, which leads to more stress and psychological disturbance, and so forth.

Fibromyalgia, like other chronic pain disorders, may require multidisciplinary treatment through specialized treatment centers: chronic pain programs or "centers of excellence." This is particularly useful for those with the most complicated psychosocial issues, including matters involving disability.

Chronic Pain Program

A chronic pain program can help people with chronic pain improve the quality of their lives. Pain symptoms and distress can be reduced, and the need to see the doctor so often can be lessened. People can gain more control over their pain. Many chronic pain multidisciplinary management programs are available throughout the country.

One approach is that developed by the Mind/Body Medical Institute at Deaconess Hospital and Harvard Medical School, under the leadership of Herbert Benson, M.D. Dr. Benson is a cardiologist and pioneer in the area of mind/body medicine. The Mind/Body Medical Institute can also direct you to a local Institute affiliated with the Mind/Body Medical Institute at Deaconess Hospital and Harvard Medical School:

The Mind/Body Medical Institute
110 Francis Street
Boston, MA 02215
(617) 632-9525
www.mindbody.harvard.edu

Relaxation audio and videotapes are available through the Mind/Body Medical Institute. The proceeds benefit the Institute.

Chronic Pain Workbook

Managing Pain Before It Manages You, by Margaret A. Caudill, M.D., Ph.D. (New York: The Guilford Press, 1995) is a pain management program in workbook form that can be used if you are not participating in a formally structured program. The program is used at the New England Deaconess Hospital in Boston, at the Hitchcock Clinic in Nashua, New Hampshire, and at Mind/Body Medical Institute affiliates around the country. Patients and health professionals in these clinics use it. It can be useful alone or when used in combination with a pain regimen prescribed by your doctor.

An Authority on Fibromyalgia Writes Personally and Professionally

Don L. Goldenberg, M.D., is Chief of Rheumatology and Director of the Arthritis/Fibromyalgia Center at Newton-Wellesley Hospital and Professor of Medicine at Tufts University School of Medicine. He is a leading authority in the area of fibromyalgia and chronic fatigue syndromes. He has written a book called *Chronic Illness and Uncertainty: A Personal and Professional Guide to Poorly Understood Syndromes* (Newton Lower Falls, MA: Dorset Press, 1996). We like this book, particularly because Dr. Goldenberg describes his personal experience with chronic pain and illness. Furthermore, he writes, "My personal reasons for writing this book include my wife's long battle with fibromyalgia. . . . I have focused much of my time and effort on fibromyalgia, since I discovered it to be the root of my own wife's struggle."

Books on Mind-Body Medicine and Healing

Another resource is Dr. Herbert Benson's excellent book, *Timeless Healing* (New York: Scribner 1996), which "explores the intersection between objective science and the mystifying power of the human spirit." Dr. Benson shows how affirming beliefs, particularly belief in a higher power, make a critical contribution to one's physical health. He advocates a balanced treatment approach that draws upon all of the elements of health care: medications, medical procedures, and self-care, including the power of the placebo response (which he calls remembered wellness).

You may wish to further explore the relationship between unconscious emotion and symptoms. We recommend *The Mindbody Prescription,* by John Sarno, M.D. (New York: Warner Books, 1998).

Centers of Excellence

Some medical centers and doctors specialize in the diagnosis and treatment of fibromyalgia. Here are several of the best specialists in fibromyalgia at major university medical centers.

Robert Bennett, M.D.
Division of Arthritis and Rheumatic
    Diseases
Oregon Health Sciences Center
3181 SW Sam Jackson Park Road
Portland, OR 97201

Don L. Goldenberg, M.D.
Director of the Arthritis/Fibromyalgia
    Center
Newton-Wellesley Hospital
2014 Washington St.
Newton, MA 02162

Frederick Wolfe, M.D.
Director, Arthritis Center
University of Kansas School of Medicine
1035 North Emporia St.
Wichita, KA 67214

John Sarno, M.D.
Professor of Clinical Rehabilitation
    Medicine
New York University Medical Center
The Rusk Institute of Rehabilitation
    Medicine
400 East 34th St.
New York, NY 10016
212-263-7300 (NYU-MC)

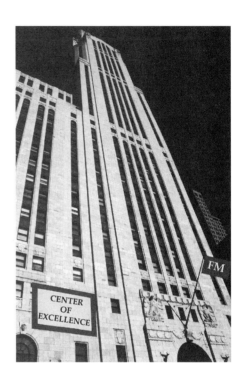

The next chapter addresses post-traumatic fibromyalgia.

Chapter 42

Post-Traumatic Fibromyalgia

Our more important role is to convince the patient that the medicolegal issues may be a negative influence on the condition (fibromyalgia) and to steer employers and lawyers to a course of rehabilitation rather than confrontation.
– Don L. Goldenberg, M.D.
(Director of the Arthritis/Fibromyalgia Center at
Newton-Wellesley Hospital and Professor of Medicine
at Tufts University School of Medicine)

Fibromyalgia can occur after an injury. Doctors call this "post-traumatic fibromyalgia." This is recognized as a legitimate medical condition by Workers' Compensation, Social Security, private insurance disability systems, and the court of law. However, because of the relative lack of objective evidence for the diagnosis of fibromyalgia, there is controversy as to whether fibromyalgia is actually caused by a specific injury or repetitive trauma.

Controversy

It is our belief that injury and repetitive trauma are just one of many factors that can contribute to the development of fibromyalgia syndrome. Although many medical and legal experts will argue that post-traumatic fibromyalgia does exist, many others will take the opposite viewpoint. The determination as to how an injured person is compensated for fibromyalgia depends upon how his (her) case is presented and argued before a hearing officer or judge. Table 42.1 compares and contrasts post-traumatic fibromyalgia from the perspective of the plaintiff and defendant.

> **Table 42.1**
>
> ## Post-Traumatic Fibromyalgia: Opposing Viewpoints
>
> | Plaintiff | Defendant |
> |---|---|
> | Diagnosis of fibromyalgia well-established | Fibromyalgia does not exist; plaintiff does not have fibromyalgia |
> | Incident (injury) clearly caused fibromyalgia | Fibromyalgia was not caused by incident (injury) |
> | Pain and disability from fibromyalgia documented and permanent | Disability minor and temporary |

Personal Injury

Post-traumatic fibromyalgia is occasionally encountered after injury or accident where a negligent party is accused. The injury usually leads to prominent symptoms and ongoing disability. Sleep disturbance and fatigue complicate the soft tissue injury, and a chronic pain condition progresses with typical symptoms and features of fibromyalgia.

What began as an innocent soft tissue injury can develop into a chronic pain condition with extensive medical care and ongoing disability. Medical bills became substantial, and treatment often becomes ineffective in healing the injury.

Personal injury cases resulting in post-traumatic fibromyalgia are usually contentious. Experts on both sides often disagree and judge and jury may determine the outcome. The legal process is stressful and may have an adverse impact upon the fibromyalgia patient.

Workers' Compensation

Proving that fibromyalgia occurred as a result of an employment accident can be difficult. A Workers' Compensation claim may be easier to resolve because the case does not rest upon whom was at fault for the injury.

Without the necessity to establish a negligent party, Workers' Compensation is more willing to allow that fibromyalgia resulted from a single event such as an accident or from cumulative or repetitive activity.

Successful Settlements

Post-traumatic fibromyalgia claims will continue to breed controversy because of the difficulty in establishing whether the incident (injury) actually caused fibromyalgia. Often, fibromyalgia results from many factors. Courts or hearing boards must determine whether a single event, such as an accident, or repetitive actions during employment was the major factor in the development of the individual's fibromyalgia.

Successful claims depend upon a clear established diagnosis. Medical records must indicate that there were no pre-existing symptoms or conditions before the accident or employment injury. Finally, it must be established that fibromyalgia was clearly the result of the accident or injury.

The next chapter addresses disability determination.

Chapter 43

Disability Determination: Workers' Compensation and Social Security

Approximately 10–20% of patients with fibromyalgia report that they are work disabled. There is much controversy regarding the medicolegal issues in such patients. Physicians should encourage such patients to continue to work, since there is evidence in many chronic pain disorders that disability adversely affects long term outcome.

– Don L. Goldenberg, M.D.
(Director of the Arthritis/Fibromyalgia Center at
Newton-Wellesley Hospital and Professor of Medicine
at Tufts University School of Medicine)

We strongly advocate that patients with fibromyalgia continue to work, especially since scientific evidence shows that disability in fibromyalgia, and in many other chronic pain disorders, adversely affects long-term outcome (e.g., satisfaction, quality of life, and comfort).

Workers' Compensation

Usually, fibromyalgia occurs independent of a work situation. But fibromyalgia can develop in association with an on-the-job injury or repetitive trauma. Thus, compensation may be allowed under the rules of the Bureau of Workers' Compensation. In order to receive benefits, the claimant will need to document several facts, including

- **A qualified physician must diagnose fibromyalgia.** The American College of Rheumatology granted official recognition of fibromyalgia

as a medical disorder in 1990.
The World Health Organization did the same in 1992.
Refer to Chapter 15 for information about diagnosis.

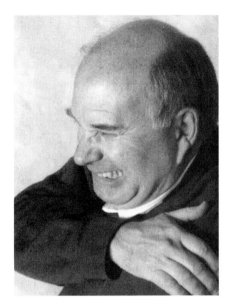

- **The date of onset of fibromyalgia must be established.**
Did it occur while the individual was employed or was it a pre-existing condition and present when the individual was hired? There can be considerable dispute as to exactly when the fibromyalgia began.

- **Unless the fibromyalgia can be associated with a specific work-related accident or event, it may be difficult to prove that the fibromyalgia was actually caused by it.**

- **The degree to which fibromyalgia has disabled the individual must be quantified.**   It is often difficult to determine and document the amount of physical impairment or disability a person experiences, especially when the physical examination and test results are normal. The physician can use the American Medical Association Guide to Permanent Impairment in order to quantify the degree of disability. In most cases, it is beneficial to the person making a claim to work with a physician who specializes in fibromyalgia.

- **A qualified doctor must provide the prognosis.**   The prognosis is the doctor's best estimate—based upon patient information, observation, and experienced clinical judgment—of how much ability the individual will be able to recover through proper treatment. The prognosis is a professional opinion based upon estimates of the duration and complexity of the disorder as well as the individual's motivation and compliance with the treatment plan.

Social Security

Qualifying for Social Security benefits related to fibromyalgia may also be difficult. As with Workers' Compensation, a person making a Social Security claim should be ready to document the existence of fibromyalgia, the date of onset of the disorder, the degree of disability experienced, and the prognosis for the individual.

However, other factors may come into play with Social Security. Advanced age may compound the effects of fibromyalgia pain and fatigue. Furthermore, education, job training, job experience, and the opportunity to pursue alternative work opportunities may figure into the resolution of a Social Security claim.

Individuals whose claims have been filed and rejected may want to seek professional advice from an attorney about appealing the rejection. An appeal guided by an attorney may bring about another case review and ultimately a change in the determination of the original claim.

In closing, we offer you one final word.

REVIEW OF STEP 7

1. Consider consulting with a doctor who specializes in fibromyalgia.

2. Other medical professionals may be able to help in your management of fibromyalgia as well.

3. Revisit the issues of stress management and dealing with emotional distress. Emotional distress can be treated, and the acceptance of emotional elements in your illness can be therapeutic.

4. If you decide to use alternative therapies or herbs, understand what you are doing. Integrate their use into a holistic *MindBodySpirit Connection* approach.

5. If necessary, consider consulting with a center of excellence or a chronic pain program.

6. Scientific evidence shows that disability in fibromyalgia, and in many other chronic pain disorders, adversely affects long-term outcome (e.g., satisfaction, quality of life, and comfort).

One Final Word

You cannot teach a man anything.
You can only help him to find it within himself.
– Galileo

> **You** are the final word because you are the healer!

This book is about you and what you can do for yourself. Knowledge is power and usually more important than medicine. You are the healer, for healing comes from within. It's up to you.

Daniel Sulmasy, M.D., a physician, ethicist, and Franciscan friar says, "All illness is multidimensional." To optimize the healing system, everyone must improve his or her health in multiple dimensions:

- Emotional—psychological
- Physical
- Social
- Spiritual

You now see that our mental state *(mind)* and physical health *(body)* are interconnected and that these connections are bidirectional. You know that the *mind* (brain) and *body* are connected through the spinal cord and nervous system and how information, including emotional information, is exchanged throughout the *mind* and *body* by way of protein chemicals called neuropeptides.

But you realize that even though chemistry is involved, your mental and emotional states can affect your physical health, and your physical health can affect your mental and emotional states. All illness like fibromyalgia has psychological and emotional consequences as well as causes. So illness is understood through a model which is both chemical *and* emotional, rather than either chemical *or* emotional.

252

Now you can appreciate the increasing evidence that *spirit* is an important part of the connection as well. *Mind* and *body* are embedded in *spirit*.

You see that *MindBodySpirit Symptoms,* like widespread musculoskeletal pain and fatigue, are experienced by all of us from time to time in one form or another. And when they bother us enough to see a doctor about them, these *MindBodySpirit Symptoms* are diagnosed as *MindBodySpirit Syndromes* like fibromyalgia. You see why so many of us experience multiple bodily symptoms and syndromes.

You understand and accept the *MindBodySpirit Connection.* We are confident that—with this knowledge and an appreciation of your own power—**you** will experience *MindBodySpirit Healing* and become stronger than you have ever been.

> **Out of the night that covers me,**
> **Black as the Pit from Pole to Pole,**
> **I thank whatever gods may be**
> **For my unconquerable soul . . .**
> **I am the master of my fate;**
> **I am the captain of my soul.**
> — *Invictus*
> William Ernest Henley

About the Authors

William B. Salt II, M.D.

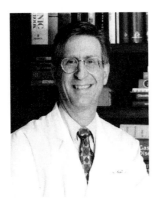

William B. Salt II, M.D., is board-certified in both internal medicine and gastroenterology. He received his M.D. degree from The Ohio State University in Columbus, Ohio, in 1972, where he currently holds an appointment as Clinical Associate Professor in Medicine. He trained for five more years in internal medicine and gastroenterology at Vanderbilt University Hospitals in Nashville, Tennessee, where he also served as a Chief Resident in Medicine.

Dr. Salt practices with the Ohio Gastroenterology Group in Columbus, Ohio. He has spent over 22 years caring for patients with digestive and liver diseases and has a special interest in irritable bowel syndrome, as well as other functional disorders. His primary hospital is Mt. Carmel Health, which is a teaching hospital and affiliate of The Ohio State University and where he serves as a chairman of the Continuing Medical Education Committee and as the Educational Director in Gastroenterology. He is actively involved in teaching medical students and residents in medicine, family practice, surgery, and obstetrics and gynecology.

His students at Mt. Carmel Health have honored him as "Teacher of the Year in Medicine, 1978–1979," and as the first nonfamily practice physician to receive the "Family Practice Residency Teacher of the Year 1995–1996." His peers have also honored Dr. Salt by including him in the fourth listing of *The Best Doctors in America*®.

The author of *Irritable Bowel Syndrome & the Mind-Body/Brain-Gut Connection,* 12 articles in medical journals, and one chapter in a book for physicians, Dr. Salt spent nearly three years collaborating with Dr. Season to write *Fibromyalgia and the MindBodySpirit Connection.* He writes, "Fibromyalgia occurs commonly with irritable bowel syndrome. These illnesses, as well as other functional bodily symptoms and syndromes, share a common origin found in the *MindBodySpirit Connection.* Understanding this is the first step to healing."

About the Authors

Edwin H. Season, M.D.

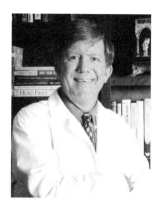 Edwin H. Season, M.D., is board-certified in orthopedic surgery. He received his M.D. degree from The Ohio State University in Columbus, Ohio, in 1971, followed by internship at the University of Virginia. He then returned to Ohio State for his residency and upon its completion, taught orthopedic surgery as an assistant professor in The Ohio State University College of Medicine from 1976 to 1980.

For the past 20 years, Dr. Season has been in the private practice of orthopedic medicine and surgery at The Ohio State University Hospitals East and Grant Medical Center in Columbus, Ohio. He is a member of the American Academy of Orthopedic Surgeons and is chairman of the Medical Advisory Committee for the State of Ohio School Employees Retirement System. He also serves on the Medical Review Board for the State of Ohio Teachers Retirement System. His special interests are fibromyalgia and musculoskeletal disability. He has participated as a medical expert in personal injury, Workers' Compensation, and Social Security hearings and deliberations.

During his years in private practice, Dr. Season has increasingly come to recognize the value of the *MindBodySpirit Connection* in his self-care, as well as its importance for his patients. He has been impressed with how his fibromyalgia patients are able to take control of their condition when they become empowered through education and improved self-care.

Dr. Season is the author of numerous scientific and medical papers that have been published in various medical journals. He collaborated with Dr. Salt for three years to write *Fibromyalgia and the MindBodySpirit Connection.* He recognizes the importance of inspiring people to heal by understanding their own power through the *MindBodySpirit Connection.*

Acknowledgments

We are extremely grateful to our friends and family who have given generously of their time and talents. Without their assistance, this work would not have been possible. First, we would like to recognize Lois Porter, our very able editor and proofreader. We can personally testify to many hours of "Conversations with Lois," via her red pen! Her meticulous perfectionism is invaluable; many thanks, Lois. Mary Ann Hopper also deserves our gratitude for excellent text design and layout. She too, is exacting in detail and always on schedule; many thanks, Mary Ann. We also thank our friend and project manager, Susan Sherron, who wears many hats, including art editor and photographer; Susan, you are the "total package!" We are especially proud and pleased to recognize our daughters, Shelley Salt and Kim Season, who have been close friends since 1st grade and who collaborated to produce the excellent line drawings in our book. Brad Salt, Dr. Salt's son, is also deserving of recognition for his exemplary skills as Web master for our Web site, which is dedicated to helping people with fibromyalgia and other functional syndromes; well done, Brad! We would also like to express appreciation to Betsy Salt for handling the Cataloging in Publication research necessary for the copyright page as well as Susan Edison for contributing to the cover design. We would also like to thank our friends at Parkview Publishing, including Michelle Brunetto, assistant project manager.

We thank our friends and colleagues who gave their valuable time to carefully read and critique the manuscript: Trenna Briscoe, Joe Brunetto, Gina Furness, Dixie Hohenadel, Rev. Tom Hudson, Carol and Doug Langenfeld, Alice McGowen, Pat Moloney, Sue Puleri, Betsy Salt, Dr. Dave Stewart, and Eileen Watkins.

We recognize and thank our cover model, Sheila Straub, for patience and professionalism. Those who also served as photographic models are Melissa Brown, Michelle Brunetto, Joe Brunetto, Kay Buckham, Connie Callif, Erin Carruthers, Rose Copp, Linda Cupp, Taneeshree Dutta, Felicia Ferst, Ruth Harris, Cynthia Kemp, Beth Leonard, Geri Martinez, Pat Moloney, Jennifer Nicol, Jessica Orlov, Sue Puleri, Earl Sagraves, Janelle Sagraves, Shelley Salt, Bob Schmitz, Linda Season, Denny Walsh, Jenny Walsh, and Barb Weber. Many thanks for your visual expressions of fibromyalgia!

Index

Notes

Notes

Notes

Notes

Visit Parkview Publishing on the Internet!

For more information on *MindBodySpirit Symptoms* and *MindBodySpirit Syndromes,* Parkview Publishing invites you to visit its Web site:

http://www.parkviewpub.com

The complete location for . . .

- Quizzes, polls, and tips
- Bulletin Board postings of your questions, tips, and experiences (hundreds of messages are posted and answered weekly)
- Real-time Chat Room, where your experiences are exchanged and shared
- Free special reports
- Fibromyalgia resources for your education and support
- "Patient to Patient"—a column authored by guest writer, Doug Langenfeld, discussing how you can successfully live with your chronic illness
- Easy, click-of-your-mouse ordering of *Fibromyalgia and the Mind-BodySpirit Connection* in electronic format (download and print it immediately at your own desk!), as well as traditional book format
- Opportunity to order other books and products related to your fibromyalgia and MindBodySpirit issues

Register your e-mail address so we can keep you updated on new products and services.

www.parkviewpub.com

Your Prescription for Change . . .

can be delivered directly to your door within three working days. Order now, and you will receive *Fibromyalgia and the MindBodySpirit Connection* for only $19.95 plus shipping and handling! If you are not completely satisfied, simply return the book at any time for a full refund, no questions asked!

To Order by Fax

Fill out the form below, including your credit card information and fax to:

Parkview Publishing
(614)-258-7272

To Order by Phone

In Columbus, Ohio: (614)-258-4848
Long distance calls (toll-free): 1-(888)-599-6464
Please have your credit card number available.

To Order by Mail

Fill out the form below and include your check (payable to Parkview Publishing), money order, or credit card information and send to:

Parkview Publishing
P.O. Box 09784
Columbus, Ohio 43209-0784

To Order by Internet

http://www.parkviewpub.com

Name _____

Address _____

City _____ State _____ Zip _____

Country _____ Phone _____

Payment method (circle one)

Personal Check   Visa   MasterCard   AMEX   Discover

Credit Card # _____ Exp date _____

Name as it appears on card _____

Within USA: $19.95 + $4.75 Shipping & Handling
Canada & Mexico: $19.95 + $9.00 Shipping & Handling
All other countries outside USA: $19.95 + $11.00 Shipping & Handling
(A list of the countries of destination is available on our Web site.)